Practice ' nd
learni isabilities

Practice Issues in Sexuality and Learning Disabilities is designed as a practical guide for all those who work in services for people with learning disabilities. It will challenge service providers to re-evaluate the implicit and explicit standards which operate in relation to sexuality and sexual expression.

Ann Craft, the editor, has an international reputation for her work on aspects of sexuality and learning disabilities, and for this book she has brought together contributions from authors in Britain, Canada and the USA. Drawing upon professional expertise from a broad range of backgrounds – social work, education, psychology, psychotherapy, medicine – the contributors tackle the practical issues and dilemmas which confront all those who work with people with learning disabilities. The contributions range from a description of the development of a statutory agency's policy document on sexuality to a carefully detailed case example of sensitive work done with pregnant women with severe learning disabilities; and from a chapter on HIV/ AIDS and safer sex counselling to a discussion of the legal position in Britain with regard to sexuality and learning disabilities. They also discuss the problems of definition and response to 'difficult' sexual behaviour, and explore the issues raised by sexual abuse.

Down-to-earth and up-to-date in its approach, the book provides practical ideas and suggestions which will be of immense value and interest to all whose work brings them into contact with people with learning disabilities – professionals, carers, parents and advocates.

Ann Craft is Senior Lecturer in the Department of Learning Disabilities, University of Nottingham Medical School.

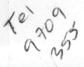

Practice issues in sexuality and learning disabilities

Edited by Ann Craft

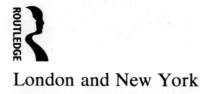

London and New York

First published 1994
by Routledge
11 New Fetter Lane, London EC4P 4EE

Simultaneously published in the USA and Canada
by Routledge
29 West 35th Street, New York, NY 10001

Typeset in Times by J&L Composition Ltd, Filey, North Yorkshire
Printed and bound in Great Britain by
TJ Press (Padstow) Ltd, Padstow, Cornwall

British Library Cataloguing in Publication Data
A catalogue record for this book is available from the British Library.

Library of Congress Cataloging in Publication Data
Practice issues in sexuality and learning disabilities/edited by Ann Craft.
    p. cm.
  Includes bibliographical references and index.
  1. Sex instruction for the mentally handicapped. 2. Mentally
handicapped–Sexual behavior. 3. Learning disabled–Sexual
behavior. I. Craft, Ann.
HQ54.3.P73   1993
306.7′087′4–dc20   93–3491
                                                                                    CIP

ISBN 0–415–05736–1 (hbk)
ISBN 0–415–05735–3 (pbk)

Contents

Contributors

Linda Andron is a Clinical Social Worker and Adjunct Lecturer in Psychiatry and Bio-Behavioral Sciences at the Neuro-Psychiatric Hospital, University of California at Los Angeles. She has been involved with services to parents with development disabilities for the past twenty years. She serves as Clinical Co-ordinator of the SHARE-UCLA Parenting Program. She has published extensively, been involved in a variety of media productions and developed curricular material. She is also involved in developing a social-relationship group treatment programme for children and young adults with autism and other social-communication disorders.

Sheila Barrett is a Lecturer/Service Development Consultant at the Centre for the Applied Psychology of Social Care at the University of Kent. She has a social work background and has worked for many years developing services and staff competencies for people with a learning disability. She has been instrumental in setting up, and currently convenes, a Diploma course in the Applied Psychology of Severe Mental Handicap (Challenging Behaviour) at the University of Kent.

Sandra Baum is a Chartered Clinical Psychologist working with people with learning disabilities, their families and support staff in London. She is also a part time lecturer at the University of East London. Her particular interests are working with adults with learning disabilities from a pychotherapeutic perspective and developing her skills in working with clients who have been sexually abused. She is the chair of RESPOND, a London-based service for people with learning disabilities who have been sexually abused.

Carol Baxter is an independent Consultant primarily concerned with equal opportunities and equity. She has written extensively in this area and has developed training materials for a number of agencies including the Department of Health. She is co-author (with Karmaljit Poonia, Linda Ward and Zenobia Nadirshaw) of *Double Discrimination – Issues and Services for People with Learning Difficulties from Black and Ethnic Minority Communities*, published by the King's Fund in 1990.

Hilary Brown is a Senior Lecturer in Learning Disabilities at the Centre for the Applied Psychology of Social Care, University of Kent. She has been concerned with sexuality issues for people with learning disabilities for many years. She has written extensively on sexuality and normalisation, and has developed many training packs including the 'Lifestyles' materials and the 'Bringing People Back Home' series of videos. She is the director of a research programme into the sexual abuse of adults with learning disabilities.

Ann Craft is a Senior Lecturer in the Department of Learning Disabilities, University of Nottingham Medical School. She has written extensively on the subject of sexuality and individuals with learning disabilities. She has developed health and sex education material for students with learning difficulties, the most recent being 'Living Your Life: A Sex Education and Personal Development Programme for Students with Severe Learning Difficulties', published by LDA in 1991. She is the co-author (with Hilary Brown) of *Working with the 'Unthinkable'* (Family Planning Association, 1992) and joint editor of *Thinking the Unthinkable* (FPA, 1989).

Thomas E. Elkins is currently Professor and Chairman of Obstetrics and Gynecology at Louisiana State University School of Medicine in New Orleans. While serving as Chief of Gynecology at the University of Michigan, he developed a model clinic for the gynecological care of persons with mental retardation, treating over 600 patients. He has published many articles related to this work, and has co-authored the book *Just Between Us: A Guide to Socialization and Sexuality* (with Dr Jean Edwards). Dr Elkins is past chairman of the Professional Advisory Board for the National Down Syndrome Congress (NDSC), a member of the NDSC Board of Directors for 9 years, and a parent of a daughter with Down's syndrome.

David Fruin is a Lecturer in the Health Services Management Unit, University of Newcastle-upon-Tyne, and is also lead officer for Community Care with Gateshead Social Services Department. He previously worked with Hertfordshire Social Services Department, developing specialist services for people with learning disabilities. As a member of a Community Health Council and a District Health

Authority, he had a special interest in improving services for people with learning disabilities.

Michael Gunn is Head of the School of Law at the University of Westminster. He has had an interest in the law as it affects people with learning disabilities for a number of years. He is author of *Sex and the Law: A Guide for Staff Working with People with Learning Disabilities* (FPA, 1991) and has written and spoken on the subject of sexuality, including sexual abuse and people with learning disabilities. He is also a member of the Mental Health Act Commission and a consultant to the Department of Health on the Mental Health Act Code of Practice.

Chris Jones is Manager at Redlands in Banbury, a day centre for adults with learning disabilities. Having trained as a clinical psychologist at the Institute of Psychiatry in London, he moved to Oxfordshire and has since worked exclusively in the field of learning disability. He has been involved directly in teaching about sexuality and personal relationships since 1978.

Michelle McCarthy and **David Thompson** work on the AIDS Awareness/Sex Education Project for people with learning difficulties, based at Harperbury Hospital. For four years they have worked full-time providing direct sex education to people with learning difficulties, staff training consultancy and policy development on HIV and sexuality issues. They have written a number of articles on the subject of sexuality and people with learning difficulties and are the authors of the recently published *Sex and the 3 R's: Rights, Responsibilities and Risks* (Pavilion Publishing, 1993).

Lorraine Millard is a freelance Trainer and Consultant working primarily in the area of sexual abuse and people with learning disabilities. She is also an individual and group therapist, specialising in work with survivors of sexual abuse and in creative therapy. Previous to this she has worked for several years as a groupworker/creative therapist with people with learning disabilities. She has been involved in the making of several training/information videos with people with learning disabilities and their carers about their lives and experiences.

John Rose is a Clinical Psychologist and Tutor on the South Wales training course in clinical psychology, based at Whitchurch Hospital, Cardiff. He has wide-ranging interests in the field of learning disabilities and has published work on topics including sexuality, staff stress, day services and consumer satisfaction.

Valerie Sinason is a Consultant Child Psychotherapist at the Tavistock Clinic and at St George's Hospital Medical School. She has specialised in the individual and group psychoanalytic psychotherapy of children and adults with learning disabilities and in the treatment of abuse victims and abusers. Her publications include *Mental Handicap and the Human Condition* (Free Association Books, 1992) and *Understanding your Handicapped Child* (Rosendale Press, 1993). She is the co-author (with Professor Shiela Hollins) of two colour picture books for abused adults with disabilities, *Jenny Speaks Out* and *Bob Tells All*. She is on the committee of VOICE and convenes the APP (Association for Psychoanalytic Psychotherapy in the NHS) Mental Handicap Section.

Dick Sobsey is a Professor in the Department of Educational Psychology at the University of Alberta in Canada. He co-ordinates the severe disabilities programme there, training teachers to work with students with severe and multiple disabilities. He is also the Director of the University of Alberta Abuse and Disability Project, a research centre dedicated to exploring the many complex relationships between abuse and disability. In addition to writing a number of books, chapters, and articles on the topics of violence and disability, he is co-author (with Fred Orelove) of *Educating Children with Multiple Handicaps: A Transdisciplinary Approach*.

David Thompson – *see* Michelle McCarthy and David Thompson above.

Alexander Tymchuk is Director of the SHARE/UCLA Parenting Program which deals specifically with parents who have a mental handicap. He is also an associate professor and is advisor to the President's Committee on Mental Retardation on parents with mental retardation. His interests deal primarily with determination on the competence and decision-making abilities of persons with mental retardation and of individuals as they age. Recently, he completed a series of studies on how persons with mental retardation make decisions about consenting to health care treatment and research participation, about entering into legal and financial contracts and into personal relationships. As part of his interest in decision-making competency, he provides evaluations of parents with mental retardation and testifies on their behalf.

Acknowledgements

The editor would like to thank Hertfordshire County Council Social Services Department for their kind permission to reproduce their Policy and Guidelines in this book.

Michael Gunn would like to point out that since his chapter of this volume; 'Compentency and consent: the importance of decision-making' was written in 1991, there have been many developments. Most notably, the Law Commission has progressed its work on Decision-Making and Mentally Incapacitated Adults, with the production of three new consultation papers: *Mentally Incapacitated Adults and Decision-Making: A New Jurisdiction* (1993, HMSO); *Mentally Incapacitated Adults and Decision-Making: Medical Treatment and Research* (1993, HMSO); and *Mentally Incapacitated and other Vulnerable Adults; Public Law Protection* (1993, HMSO). That chapter should be read in the light of the contribution these papers make to the debate discussed therein, and in the light of the developments indicated therein.

1 Personal relationships and sexuality
The staff role

Ann Craft and Hilary Brown

INTRODUCTION

Whether members of staff are conscious of it or not, they play a central part in the personal relationship needs of people with a learning disability. They are inevitably drawn into a form of intimacy, in physical caring, in emotional responsiveness, in social activities and networks, which has no obvious parallel. To meet the demands placed on them they may draw on a range of models to guide them about appropriate involvement and boundaries, they may base their relationships on those they have with their children or siblings, with friends or colleagues, or on more established 'professional' roles such as that of a teacher, counsellor or social worker. Any of these may be valid, in whole or in part, but all imply different approaches to:

— goals of intervention
— style of work
— expertise and knowledge
— appropriate distance
— mix of control and empowerment
— accountability and openness.

By looking more closely at what these roles involve it is hoped that we can delineate a distinctive mode of working on sexuality issues, which enables staff to be more purposeful and empowering in their work with individuals with a learning disability.

The chapter has three main sections. First we will look at the general context of professional interactions between staff and individuals with a learning disability. Second we shall explore the various aspects of a positive staff role in relation to the personal relationships and sexuality needs of service users. Third, we will consider the needs of staff if they are to fulfil this positive role.

THE CONTEXT OF STAFF/SERVICE USER RELATIONSHIPS

Before looking specifically at the staff role in relation to client needs in the area of personal relationships and sexuality, we need to look at the general context in which professional staff interact with clients who have learning disabilities. As Brechin and Swain (1988) point out in their thoughtful analysis, 'Relationships between professionals and people labelled as having a mental handicap have their origins in past and present social structures and attitudes'. The authors characterise and describe the two main approaches to people with learning difficulties which have been prominent in the past fifty years – the medical approach and the educational approach. Both approaches:

> assume that existing social constructions of normality define the goal to which people with learning difficulties must aspire; both define and understand the 'problems of mentally handicapped' people in such a way as to indicate clearly the impossibility of ever achieving that goal (the best hope being to build up patterns of skills which approximate to 'normal' behaviour); and both create a professional/client relationship which enshrines the professional in a world of exclusive and privileged knowledge, and consequently entombs the individual with learning difficulties in a fundamentally dependent role.
>
> (Brechin and Swain 1988)

Brechin and Swain suggest that the aims of the comparatively recent self-advocacy movement, with its emphasis on self-actualisation and an open-ended process of growth, can be used 'as a kind of litmus test of appropriateness against which professional approaches can be measured'. Their outline for shared action planning (Brechin and Swain 1987) is an attempt to foster partnership, to build up a 'working alliance' (Deffenbacher 1985).

In conclusion, Brechin and Swain (1988) suggest that from the perspective of people with learning disabilities, a working alliance with professionals should seem:

— to be an entitlement rather than an imposition
— to promote self-realisation rather than compliance
— to open up choices rather than replace one option with another
— to develop opportunities, relationships and patterns of living, in line with their individual wishes rather than rule-of-thumb normality
— to enhance their decision-making control of their own lives
— to allow them to move at their own pace.

Each of these six points has relevance when we consider the personal relationship and sexuality needs of individuals with a learning disability and the way in which services and members of staff respond to them.

An important part of this context of staff/service user relationships is the 'increasing tendency to articulate a set of principles setting out what are believed to be the "rights" of clients' (Hudson 1988). Craft (1987) suggests six rights pertaining to sexuality:

— the right to grow up, i.e. to be treated with the respect and dignity accorded to adults
— the right to know, i.e. to have access to as much information about themselves and their bodies and those of other people, their emotions, appropriate social behaviour, etc. as they can assimilate
— the right to be sexual and to make and break relationships
— the right not to be at the mercy of the individual sexual attitudes of different care-givers
— the right not to be sexually abused
— the right to humane and dignified environments.

However, because of the nature of intellectual disability, societal attitudes and the structure of services, many individuals with learning disabilities require some degree of help and assistance in exercising those (and other) rights. This enabling process may take place at different levels, ranging from one-to-one counselling to the adoption of policy guidelines across a whole service.

THE STAFF ROLE

Staff members as role models

Whether staff members like it or not, whether they acknowledge it or not, they are enormously powerful in the lives of people with learning disabilities. Powerful in terms of the physical environments that are provided in day and residential services; powerful in terms of the social environments that they create; powerful in the spoken and unspoken feedback they give about client aspirations and behaviour; and powerful in offering models of adult men and women with adult lifestyles making adult choices (Bandura 1977).

Much of the modelling is at a very informal level. Nevertheless it has strong influences on many of the people with whom staff members come into contact. The way that managers interact with staff, staff with colleagues, with people with a learning disability, the way that staff members show pleasure, anger, approval, disapproval, that they are upset, that they are having an off day, all give messages to others. Do members of staff model respect for the feelings and attitudes of others in the way that they talk to them? Do they respect people's need for space and privacy? Does the language they use accord dignity to people? Is it age-appropriate? The danger is that staff members' way of relating gives the message, 'do as I say, not as I do'. Implicitly staff may model one way of interacting with others, while explicitly they are telling those others that they should behave in a different way.

As in the example below, some of the models of adult interaction offered by members of staff can be a source of confusion and frustration to individuals with learning disabilities.

Gerald, a man with moderate learning disabilities, had recently moved from a hospital setting to a group home. After a few months staff asked for help in managing Gerald's 'aggressive outbursts'. On one occasion he had broken the windscreen wipers on a visitor's car, on another he had smashed the same car's headlights. He had also pulled his key worker's hair and threatened to punch her when she remonstrated with him for giving her a bonecrushing hug.

On investigation it transpired that Gerald, coming from a male hospital ward with male staff, was convinced that his female key worker's enthusiastic involvement in his progress and wellbeing was a sign of sexual interest. This misapprehension had been fostered unthinkingly by other members of staff, who at first jokingly agreed with Gerald when he referred to his key worker as his 'girlfriend', then actively promoted by teasing remarks such as, 'poor Gerald, your girlfriend's not here today'.

Gerald's key worker was inexperienced. She had not challenged Gerald's early references to her as 'my girlfriend'. As she said, 'I didn't think there was any harm in it, and he looked so pleased to see me I didn't want to spoil the relationship I was building with him'. Similarly, although she later commented that Gerald's physical approaches increasingly made her feel uncomfortable, she had not objected at first because she knew how emotionally impoverished his life in the hospital had been. The damaged car belonged to the key worker's boyfriend, understandably seen by Gerald as a rival for her affection.

Gerald, with few models to draw upon, was for a time confirmed in his beliefs by the explicit validation and repetition of his verbal claims, and by the acceptance of physical touch. Staff chose to amuse themselves with what they saw as 'only harmless teasing';

Gerald's key worker allowed her boundaries of personal space to be invaded on the mistaken assumption that she was somehow compensating for past deprivation, and that this and the joking remarks were justifiable because they increased the rapport she needed to establish as a good key worker.

While members of staff and the key worker were all clear in their own minds where the boundaries lay – that Gerald was not, and would never be her boyfriend – Gerald had no means of knowing this. The seemingly abrupt volte-face by his key worker and the disapproval of other staff when their limits of tolerance were reached confused and upset Gerald. It required careful reappraisal on everyone's part to arrive at acceptable boundaries of language and touch. Gerald paid an unacceptably high price in terms of his mental health, his self esteem and self confidence.

It is not only personal boundaries which can become confused in this way but more diffuse gender expectations and roles may be passed onto people with learning disabilities in contradictory ways. Despite equal opportunities statements and commitments, services on the whole replicate patterns of inequality within the home, with their predominantly female workforce but male management. Men with learning disabilities are thus offered role models of men 'in charge', who are able to command respect and use their status with the women who are employed as care staff, while they themselves are 'under' the control of those women. Men with learning disabilities react differentially to staff depending on their place in the hierarchy. Brown and Ferns (1991) filmed a black woman who reported an incident in which a resident had taken advice from a male care worker and from a white woman who was a deputy manager, but ignored her input. These issues are difficult to acknowledge but important. This man, while his behaviour, being racist and sexist, is unacceptable, is perhaps also trying to find out where *he* stands in the hierarchy, and how he *can* legitimately assert himself as a man in the way that he sees other men assert themselves.

Services may also pass on roles and expectations which are at odds with learned patterns of behaviour within service users' families and within their wider religious or cultural communities. 'Unisex' attitudes, which tend to prevail in mixed group homes, may jar with people who come from families which have fairly prescribed and *different* roles, rules and responsibilities for men and women. Helping men and women reach an acceptable compromise between traditional values and new or unfamiliar roles is something which requires adaptability and sensitivity on the part of staff rather than dogmatic and sometimes ill-informed idealism. In creating an environment in which men and women with learning disabilities can express 'gender' as well as sexuality, staff need to be aware of the backgrounds of the people who use the service and of the impact men and women's roles in either family or service environments have had on their skills, interests and aspirations.

Staff as teachers

Staff may work with individuals with learning disabilities in a number of contexts. Providing a member of staff is competent in, and feels comfortable with, setting up and running structured programmes covering personal relationships and sexuality, that person is in an ideal position to do so. She or he will know the students in the group well, and will have an understanding of individual needs. However, it should not be assumed that everyone will be comfortable with the more formal teaching role (see the section on training, p. 19).

There are now a number of teaching resources available, many specifically designed for students with learning disabilities, which offer an overall structure of personal, social and sexual education. See for example Brook Advisory Centres 1987; Craft and Members of the Nottinghamshire SLD Sex Education Project 1991; Dixon 1992; Dixon and Craft 1992; Craft, 1992. Each of these packs or programmes provides flexibility, so that the needs of individual students or groups can be accommodated.

Staff do not only have a role in setting up and running structured education programmes, but also, and very importantly, in responding to what educationalists call 'the teachable moment'. This is when an opportunity to teach arises naturally from a situation or event. For example, when a person with a learning disability asks a particular question, or shows evidence of confusion about behaviour which is acceptable in private, but not in public. For staff members to feel comfortable with this aspect of their role they need policy guidelines and support from senior management (see section on staff needs below).

Staff as counsellors

Whether or not an establishment has a structured programme on personal relationships, some people with learning disabilities will need individual or pair counselling about aspects of their lives. Again, some staff members will not want to see themselves as counsellors, and others, who in principle would be interested to develop their skills in this area, need training opportunities to do so.

The need for counselling about personal relationships and sexuality can be seen at a number of different levels. The PLISSIT model offers a helpful way of looking at these levels (Annon 1974). PLISSIT stands for different levels of counselling and intervention: *P*ermission, *L*imited *I*nformation, *S*pecific *S*uggestions and *I*ntensive *T*herapy. The model posits a decreasing number of clients at each of the levels, with the majority of people presenting for counselling only requiring the first level – permission giving. At this level the counsellor, by the non-judgemental and reassuring approach adopted, 'allows' the client to engage in behaviours in which they are already engaging, but which they think are abnormal; or gives permission to engage in behaviours they have been avoiding. When we think about people with learning disabilities, often the 'permission giving' has to include their parents and care staff in helping them to understand that it is to be expected, not abnormal, for such individuals to have sexual feelings and to want to give expression to those feelings. Moreover, for people with learning disabilities this permission giving may have to overturn previous, sometimes explicit 'prohibitions' arising from negative feedback and imagery. People with learning disabilities will sometimes be heard verbally admonishing themselves for their own sexual behaviour as they give voice to the previously unchallenged disapproval of those around them. Indeed there is evidence that as a group they have internalised attitudes about sexuality which are more conservative and negative than those of other people (Watson and Rogers 1980a, 1980b; Brantlinger 1985).

A smaller number of people will need more than permission giving and will require limited information directly related to their sexual concerns. A decreasing number of clients will require specific suggestions, with the counselling assisting them to set and reach goals. The final level of intensive therapy is needed by the least number of clients, but is the most serious and is likely to be long term rather than the relatively brief intervention at the other three levels. Intensive therapy requires a high degree of professional competence and should *not* be attempted by anyone who has not undertaken supervised training in sexual counselling.

This hierarchy is helpful to keep in mind because it signals that besides different levels of client need, there are also different degrees of professional competence needed. No staff member should be pressured to undertake work beyond what they feel is their level of competence. Sometimes staff fall (or get pushed) into the trap of believing that they should be able to answer every single question, be able to deal with every single difficulty or anxiety presented by the person with a learning disability. It is important to be clear that it is a very legitimate and professional position to recognise and acknowledge that there will be limits to everyone's expertise and individual members of staff should not be pressured into work that goes beyond that point. It should in no way be seen as a failure when a staff member engaged in counselling comes to a point when they need to ask for help themselves, or to refer the client on. Indeed, counsellors should have access to a supportive supervision system within which such concerns can be aired.

Liaising with other professionals and/or with parents

This will not be the role of every staff member, but in each setting it should be clear whose responsibility it is to do that liaison work. All too often day and residential services operate in isolation from each other, to the detriment of the person with a learning disability who moves between both.

Part of this role will be acting as a 'broker' – bringing in or buying in services to meet people's needs. A prerequisite for doing this is to build up a network list of local resource people and services. For example, Health Education Units (see under your Health Authority in the phone book) are often useful sources of sex education teaching materials; RELATE may be able to suggest a counsellor or sex therapist; local Brook or family planning clinics may welcome organised visits; the HIV/AIDS Education Officer will have up-to-date information and may help with individual work or teaching (for example, over the course of a year in one Nottingham school for pupils with severe learning difficulties, the HIV/AIDS Education Officer came in regularly to work with older students, and run seminars for staff and a much-welcomed workshop for parents).

Where links on behalf of clients are attempted with generic services an important feature of the liaison role is to help professionals in those services to develop confidence and competence in working with people with learning disabilities. All too often the first response from those in a generic service is likely to be an inclination to exclude individuals on the grounds that their service is not designed for people with learning disabilities; the presence of a learning disability means that the person would not be able to benefit from the service; nothing in their professional training prepared them for working with such clients and they would not know where to start. However, there are ways of overcoming these hurdles. For example, it is helpful to make links with generic colleagues to discuss the possibility of any future referrals. This could be with staff at your local family planning clinic or with the Rape Crisis Centre team. You can also explore opportunities for joint working, bringing together a professional from services for people with learning disabilities and a generic specialist, each pooling ideas and strategies drawn from their own experience and training. It might be possible to set up sessions of counselling or psychotherapy for a client, jointly supervised by a professional from a generic service and one from the specialist service (Craft and Slack, in press). Fundamentally, the needs of people with learning disabilities are far more similar to those of the rest the population than they are different, and many, if not all, of the strategies and approaches used by professionals in generic services will be applicable. Working in tandem can enable you to plan any adaptations which may be needed.

In liaison work, staff need to show sensitivity towards the anxieties of parents. Parents have very real concerns about the perceived vulnerability of their daughters and sons (Brown 1987). The parents of adults may never have had the chance to be supported in thinking through the implications of their offspring as sexual beings with physical and emotional needs. There are welcome signs that more and more schools are now working with parents along these lines (Craft and Cromby 1991) but it is rarer for the parents of adults to have such opportunities. However, some helpful models do exist. See for example chapter two by Rose and Jones in this book; Lewisham Special Needs Sexuality Project (1988); Open University (1986).

Staff as protectors

As a group, individuals with learning disabilities are likely to have increased vulnerability to sexual exploitation and abuse (see chapter five in this book by Sobsey; Turk and Brown 1992)). Management and staff have a responsibility towards the personal integrity and safety of individuals with learning difficulties within care systems. Walmsley (1989) offers an analysis of the ways in which the organisation and delivery of services can enhance or decrease protection, and in his chapter in this book (chapter five), Sobsey shows how the ethos of an establishment can shape or 'license' staff behaviour that is exploitative or abusive.

We have referred to policy documents on the personal relationships and sexuality of individuals with learning disabilities. Another welcome trend is the development of procedural guidelines on service responses to the abuse or vulnerability of adults (Nottingham Health Authority and Nottinghamshire Social Services Department 1992; ADSS 1991; Brown and Stein, in preparation). The existence of guidelines puts the subject onto the official agenda of services, and also spells out individual staff members' responsibilities (see note at end of chapter on NAPSAC, and Brown and Craft, in preparation).

However, many dilemmas facing staff hover on the borders of definitions of exploitation and abuse. Where service users with differing degrees of intellectual and physical disability interact it is often open to individual and arbitrary interpretation whether one person with a learning disability is exploiting another. Brown and Turk (1992) help us explore the dimensions involved in the concepts of abuse and consent. As Gunn points out in chapter six, the issue of capacity to consent is a thorny one. Where one or both parties has a severe learning disability and therefore capacity to consent is debatable (see Gunn 1991), Figure 1.1 offers an approach which can clarify decisions and remove them from the domain of the individual staff member. (See also the role play exercise entitled 'We'd Better Call a Case Conference' in Brown and Craft 1992 which reminds us that different interested parties will have different agendas.) We suggest that the relationship or encounter giving rise to concern is analysed separately for each party, as it is important not to muddle their needs, intentions and impact on each other.

Figure 1.1   Exploitation or not?

(Use this form separately for *each* of the parties concerned)

Definition

- What is the behaviour which is causing concern (afterwards referred to as 'behaviour under review')? Be as precise as possible, ie.:
  — what can you see happening?
  — what are you afraid might be happening behind closed doors?
- Who is involved?
- What makes you think that the person you are concerned about is:
  — in distress
  — in need of protection
  — in need of intervention?
- Do you think that the person is under pressure:
  — physically
  — sexually
  — emotionally
  — financially?

- Has the behaviour under review begun recently, or does it have a long history?
- How frequently does it occur?
- What happens before/after the behaviour under review?

Background

- Under ordinary circumstances, how does the person you are concerned about usually indicate pleasure/distress?
  e.g. — smiles, claps hands when parents arrive to take her/him out
       — becomes withdrawn and moody, sleep disturbed when upset.
  (Different staff may pick up different cues, so check with as many staff as possible.)
- Under other circumstances, how does the person you are concerned about protect her/himself or resist things they do not want to happen?
  e.g. — makes high-pitched noise, resists physical prompts by running off or kicking out when s/he does not want to come in from the garden.
- Has this person had, or do they have, similar relationships/encounters with a number of other people?
- How does the person you are concerned about usually get on with the other person? Record views of different staff members.
  e.g. — one party ignore other(s) except when s/he wants to engage in the behaviour under review
       — often seek out each other's company.
- Has the person you are concerned about ever complained about the behaviour of the other(s) involved in the behaviour under review? Under what circumstances?
- Following the behaviour under review, has any physical harm to the person been recorded?
- Following the behaviour under review, do any of the parties concerned show signs of pleasure/disress? What are these signs?

Discussion

- What do you and your colleagues think are the advantages/disadvantages of the behaviour under review to the person concerned?

Recommendations

- Following information-gathering and discussions, what recommendations do you now wish to make?

Review

- Does the implementation of the recommendations need to be reviewed? If so, set a date to do this.

With sexual abuse staff clearly have a protective role to play. In other circumstances it is tempting for staff to steer either for the Scylla of over-protectiveness (where they actively, but unrealistically, attempt to prevent *any* emotional upset befalling service users) or the

Charybdis of *laissez-faire* (where nearly all forms of sexual risk-taking and expression are mistakenly seen as part of normalisation). Neither position is helpful to those with learning disabilities. Personal and sexual relationships have the potential for pain and heartbreak as well as pleasure; that is an integral part of the human condition. Some risks are necessary for learning and personal growth. At the other extreme, there is no comparable degree of risk-taking between, for example, a man without a learning disability who knows about safer sex but chooses on occasion not to wear a condom, and a man with a learning disability who knows little or nothing about HIV, little or nothing about condoms or how to put one on. Similarly, a woman with a learning disability, encouraged all her life to do as she is told, with little sense of personal danger, is engaging in risk through ignorance, not choice, if she agrees to go home with the man who picks her up at the disco. There *is* a path between over- and under-protection of service users. It will be a different path for different individuals, but the process of delineating it should be guided by service principles of good practice rather than be left up to one member of staff. Carson (1992) suggests that it would often be appropriate to subject any 'proposed intervention to a risk analysis, to ensure that the expected benefits sufficiently outweigh the anticipated harms'.

Staff as interveners

Where a particular sexual behaviour brings a person with learning disabilities into conflict with legal and societal boundaries, it may be necessary for staff to intervene. Indeed, as Carson (1992) asks, could service providers be seen as negligent for *not* intervening?

> If a client regularly behaves in a socially inappropriate manner, for example, exposing himself in public, then his participation in the community and enjoyment of it, is likely to be reduced. He is experiencing a significant loss. Failing to do something, to help this individual behave in a lawful and more socially acceptable manner, is not a neutral or a safe option for service providers.
>
> (Carson 1992)

Carson goes on to spell out how an intervention process should be developed in ways that are consistent with standards of good professional practice.

Shelton (1992) describes a carefully monitored intervention to help a man with profound learning disabilities learn a masturbation technique which increased his low rate of ejaculation and decreased his high risk of self-injury. Mitchell (1985) offers a behavioural approach to interventions relating to sexual activity, which emphasises the importance of careful recording and clarity of definitions. Brown and Barrett in their chapter in this book (chapter three) help us tease out the complexities involved in what we label 'difficult sexual behaviour'.

Any intervention which aims at reshaping sexual behaviour should be carefully considered and planned. It should also be well documented, with clear reference to who is responsible for doing what, under what circumstances, over what time period and with what monitoring and evaluation. Crisis situations may require swift on-the-spot response, but no individual member of staff should take it upon her or himself to instigate a longer-term intervention relating to a client's sexual behaviour without the official sanction and support of the staff team, arrived at through the consultation process.

Staff as advocates and supporters of self-advocacy

In many areas, not least among them personal relationships and sexuality, a staff member may find themselves speaking up for people who, for a variety of reasons, are not able to speak powerfully or effectively on their own behalf. This may be to representatives of the management structure, to colleagues or to an individual's parents. The existence of policy guidelines relating to sexuality and individuals with learning disabilities can facilitate this role as the policy is likely to have clearly articulated individual rights (see section above on the context of staff/service user relationships and chapter thirteen by Fruin). These rights may need to be translated into the everyday operation of services. For example, what is the forum for discussing and reaching decisions about an individual client's needs in relation to his or her personal relationships and expressions of sexuality? Is it an automatic part of the IPP or review process (Jones *et al.* 1991)? If so, how is confidentiality guarded? If not, how do such issues get onto the agenda in a way that is not solely a response to a 'problem' or a 'crisis'? In any review, how are the religious and cultural dimensions of the person's life taken into account?

In recent years there has been a growth of local self-advocacy initiatives (EMFEC 1991; Whittaker 1991). These implicitly and explicitly encourage exploration of a sense of personhood – Who am I? How am I the same as others, how am I different? What do I like/dislike? What do I want? How do I ask for what I want? How can I achieve what I want without stopping others from doing what they want? How do I see my future? There has also been an increase in opportunities to explore what it means to be a woman or a man with the label of 'learning disability' in women's or men's groups (see for example the videotape *Between Ourselves*). Any work done on self-awareness, personal integrity, decision-making, adulthood, relation-ships and sexuality inevitably spills out beyond the confines of the learning context into other areas of people's lives. This is something to be nurtured.

However, if people with learning disabilities exercise more power, someone has to relinquish it – this may be the staff, it may be parents. It is not easy to do. Here we touch upon central questions of control, of protection, of best interests, of responsibilities. It moves us into the area of risk-taking, never an easy nettle to grasp, for staff or for parents. Power is very one-sided within most service structures – this makes it difficult for staff members to 'hear' or to treat seriously aspirations of service users which do not fit, which threaten to upset the system, which challenge a staff member's sense of their own role as someone 'in charge', who 'knows best'. But, as Brechin and Swain (1988) tell us:

> Self-advocacy is in essence about a process of self-actualisation. It is about people coming to identify and express personal feelings, wishes and circumstances and coming to understand what contributes to the positives and negatives of their existence. It is about opening up ideas about the range of choices which could and should be available to them.
>
> Any professional approach that does not concern itself with supporting and facilitating these same processes of growth for people with learning difficulties must be seriously open to question. Similarly, approaches which seem to imply a pre-knowledge of the aims and goals of other people's lives, and lack the willingness to retain an open mind, to live with uncertainties, possibilities and transitions – these too must be seen as professional approaches with little to recommend them.
>
> (Brechin and Swain 1988)

Staff as empowerers

This sums up the staff role. It is about enabling individuals by a process of encouragement, facilitation and the imparting of skills to exercise power over their own lives and to make their own choices at their own pace.

The process of support has to be an active one, for as Brechin and Swain (1988) point out:

> It is too simplistic to suggest that by offering improved opportunities in a less restrictive setting, individuals with often severe learning difficulties, frequently additional disabilities, and histories of damaging experience, will thereby have *access* to improved, more satisfying life-styles. Access requires more than just the existence of possibilities.

Within the context of this chapter – personal relationships and sexuality – this means that:

— individuals with learning disabilities are encouraged to learn as much as they can about their physical growth and development, their emotions, themselves as sexual beings, risks and consequences
— opportunities for a rich social life are actively pursued with them and on their behalf
— individual sexual needs are addressed within an agreed professional structure which has a built-in partnership with the person concerned
— individual sexual needs are responded to in ways which accord dignity and respect and which take into account the person's religious and cultural values
— counselling services are readily available and accessible
— service delivery is guided by a written policy within which individual rights to privacy etc. are clearly delineated.

STAFF NEEDS

In order to take on the multifaceted role outlined above, members of staff themselves need an enabling structure within which to operate.

Managing the tension arising from ambiguities

In seeking to define a helpful stance for workers in relation to sexuality, managers of services need to be aware of conflicts at several levels. Individual staff members may shift from one role to another as the situation dictates, or in response to their own mood, experience or prejudices. They may for example be very facilitative to hetero-sexual couples who have agreed not to have children but act in a punitive way to same sex couples, or to partners who want to be parents. They may hover between being protective and taking a *laissez-faire* stance. There will also be differences within staff teams which, if managed well, enable group decisions to be more objective and balanced than judgements made in isolation. If conflicting views can be made explicit and respected (even if disagreed with) they can provide additional safeguards to those service users on whose behalf decisions are being made and/or services are being delivered.

There may also be inconsistencies within the wider organisation, for example, liberal policies undermined by prohibitive resource decisions, or half-hearted support for empowering service users which is withdrawn at the first high profile decision which is contentious. Local politicians, lay management boards and the community at large may all put a restraining influence on senior managers.

Parents' groups may also seek to restrain and are often polarised from staff for many reasons (Brown 1987). The protective response they seek from staff may stem, in part, from their experience of the community's ambivalence to their sons and daughters and their more cautious approach to independence reflects their day-to-day contact with, and often responsibility for, the person's dependency needs.

Against this background it is easy to see why sexuality is a contentious issue and a cause of stress to staff. This stress which is often characterised as personal 'up tightness' has its roots in the organisation's inability to clarify a coherent agenda around sexuality issues. However clear the agency's explicit values with reference to supporting people with learning disabilities in seeking positive sexual options, there may also be a pull towards conservatism which is mirrored in the behaviour of individual staff.

It is important to clarify this divergence since it creates a tendency for services to become paralysed and to 'split off' opposing views. These splits fragment services' input along emotive 'fracture' lines with different stakeholders polarised on either bank. Permissiveness v. protection, staff v. parents, victim v. perpetrator, the list of false choices could go on. The reality is that services, if they are to square the circle, have to provide both protection and sensitive opportunities, they have to work with people who have been abused and with those who abuse others (sometimes in the same person, let alone service), they have to find ways not of excluding families but of bringing them in on the task of supporting adulthood and adult options.

Thus the real choice for services is not along those particular fault lines but about the extent to which they *actively* support and empower service users in their personal and sexual lives. Most services avoid difficult issues by 'lying low' and hoping nothing happens. Such an approach almost guarantees that nothing will happen, or that if it does it will be met with a 'containing' rather than empowering reaction. Sadly, this is as true of dealing with positive sexual relationships as with difficult sexual behaviour.

Sexuality, in effect, becomes a source of immense stress for staff whose personal values and professional skills jostle for place in this organisational vortex. An understanding of the sources of this stress will help staff towards a more appropriate role. Organisational analysts identify two kinds of stress where roles are problematical. 'Role ambiguity' is the technical term for the kind of personal discomfort wherein individuals are uncomfortable about the role they are being asked to perform. 'Role conflict' describes the position of staff being asked to undertake incompatible tasks or roles, in situations where explicit aims are not consistent with unspoken agendas and where the result is confused expectations. Both of these situations are accurate predictors of staff stress, dissatisfaction and turnover (Handy 1976; Jackson and Schuler 1985). Both are common in relation to sexuality.

Policy guidelines

It is against this background that policy guidelines have to be formulated. As well as informing staff, guidelines work to put limits on role ambiguity and role conflict. Early guidelines such as those from Hounslow (1982) acknowledge the problem of role ambiguity and later guidelines develop the point and reassure staff that they will not be asked to be involved beyond a threshold of personal tolerance:

> There are no doubt aspects of these guidelines which, on the basis of their own ethical or moral code, some staff might disagree with or find personally unacceptable. It should therefore be stated that there is no expectation that they should change their own standards. Equally, however they would not be expected, as professionals, to impose these standards upon their clients.
>
> (Hounslow Social Services Department 1982)

Reaching an understanding of the sexual needs of someone with a learning disability is difficult for care givers. This is so because we are now coming to understand that it is simply not good enough either to ignore the issue or to respond only when and if an individual begins to act in overtly sexual ways. As the Social Services Committee statement puts it, there is recognition of '**the rights of adults with mental handicaps to understand, develop and express their sexuality**' within certain limits. Your role is more than, and subtly different from, the role of a friend or an outside advocate; it encompasses a specific duty to act, as an aspect of your professional task.

You may have definite views yourself about what is right and wrong in sexual matters, but at work you should be guided by this recognition.

(East Sussex County Council 1992, emphasis in the original)

Guidelines should thus attempt to outline a role which is consistently proactive and supportive, one which is 'professional' in the sense that it has proper boundaries and accountability built in and one which is consistent with the philosophy of the service. By assuring staff that they do *not* have to be all things to all people, that, if they have used appropriate consultation procedures, they do not have to carry all the risks alone, guidelines should help staff to deal with role ambiguity.

A recent conceptualisation of job related stress is one set out by Karasek and Theorell (1990) which looks at jobs in terms of the level of psychological demands they present and the scope for decision-making and autonomy. Active jobs which incorporate a high degree of control tend to lead to 'healthy stress', whereas those in demanding jobs in which people have less control over decision-making run the greatest risk of psychological or physical ill effects. Since sexual issues, and care work in general, are inherently demanding we can see that a key function of guidelines must be to define the greatest possible leeway within which individual workers and teams can reach their own decisions. While stress is often characterised as the province of high-flying decision-makers, Karasek and Theorell are unequivocal that 'It is the bossed, not the bosses who experience most stress in our society . . .' and that it is 'constraints on decision making, not decision making per se which is the major problem for most workers'.

Guidelines then have two functions, to draw some acceptable boundary around the personal and the professional and to define the boundaries within which individual workers can respond as they think best. Since increased decision-making is the aim, training and information must be made available to equip front-line staff with the skills and knowledge they need to act authoritatively both on behalf of, and sometimes in relation to, service users.

Periodic formal reviews of policy documents can be the forum to re-evaluate practice, and should be an important feature of service organisation.

Training

Training is absolutely essential if staff are to be enabled to carry out the roles we have discussed. Training has to be on at least two levels. All staff need an *awareness* training – awareness that individuals with an intellectual disability have needs and rights in relation to their sexuality. They also need *information* on a range of issues such as local services, educational resources available, HIV transmission, pregnancy and so on. Such training can be given as part of an induction course or part of in-service work.

At a second level, some, but not all staff, will wish to undertake further training so that they can become the teachers and the counsellors. Such courses, if not available locally, can be had from a variety of national organisations, for example, the British Institute of Learning Disabilities (BILD); the Association to Aid the Personal and Sexual Relationships of People with Disabilities (SPOD); the Education and Training Department of the Family Planning Association; Brook Advisory Centres, Birmingham.

Support

The support offered to staff by the existence of policy guidelines has already been mentioned. With the acceptance of such guidelines should come support from managers for staff working within the established procedures (Brown and Ferns 1991).

Not everyone in a particular setting will be involved in formal teaching or in counselling, but those who are should be able to receive support from colleagues, so that their work is not undermined. For this to happen there needs to be a system of feedback which does not sacrifice confidentiality, but which allows non-involved staff to be aware that counselling is still in progress, or that the sex education group has reached a particular point in the agreed curriculum.

An important source of support is via monitoring and evaluation. This can be on an informal basis, for instance by the co-teachers of a sex education group setting aside a regular time to reflect on the teaching session; or more formally, where for instance, a counsellor receives supervision from a qualified person.

In a number of areas people who work in different services for people with learning disabilities have formed a special interest group focusing on issues relating to sexuality and personal relationships. Such a group can fulfil several purposes – it brings staff members into contact with other supportive and concerned professionals; it offers a forum for discussing dilemmas, for reviewing new resources and for sharing ideas about good practice.

CONCLUSION

In this chapter we have attempted to define the different roles staff have to play in response to the personal relationships and sexuality needs of people with learning disabilities. These roles are played out against the background of the tenor and tone of professional interactions between members of staff and individuals with learning disabilities, and in the general context of the ethos of service organisations. As we went on to explore, the sexuality of service users throws up particular challenges, ambiguities and tensions both for individual staff members and for services as a whole. Policy guidelines, training and support are all required to enable staff to act positively, constructively and responsibly in response to the individual sexual needs of people with learning disabilities.

NOTE

NAPSAC (the National Association for the Protection from Sexual Abuse of Adults and Children with Learning Disabilities) is an information network for professionals and agencies. For further information contact NAPSAC Development Officer, Department of Learning Disabilities, University of Nottingham Medical School, Queens Medical Centre, Nottingham NG7 2UH.

REFERENCES

ADSS (Association of Directors of Social Services) (1991) *Adults at Risk: Guidance for Directors of Social Services*. London: ADSS.

Annon, J. (1974) *The Behavioral Treatment of Sexual Problems*, Vol. 1: *Brief Therapy*, Honolulu: Enabling Systems.

Bandura, A. (1977) *Social Learning Theory*. New Jersey: Prentice Hall.

Between Ourselves (1988) 15-minute video for purchase or hire, Twentieth Century Vixen, 28 Southampton Street, Brighton, East Sussex BN2 2UT.

Brantlinger, E. (1985) 'Mildly mentally retarded secondary students' information about and attitudes toward sexuality and sexuality education', *Education and Training of the Mentally Retarded* June: 99–108.

Brechin, A. and Swain, J. (1987) *Changing Relationships: shared action planning with people with a mental handicap*. London: Harper & Row.

Brechin, A. and Swain, J. (1988) 'Professional/client relationships: creating a "working alliance" with people with learning difficulties'. *Disability, Handicap & Society* 3 (3): 213–26.

Brook Advisory Centres (1987) *Not A Child Anymore*. Birmingham: Brook Advisory Centres.

Brown, H. (1987) 'Working with parents', in Craft, A. (ed.) *Mental Handicap and Sexuality: Issues and Perspectives*. Tunbridge Wells: Costello.

Brown, H. and Craft, A. (1992) *Working with the 'Unthinkable': A staff training pack on the sexual abuse of adults with learning difficulties*. London: Family Planning Association.

Brown, H. and Craft, A. (in preparation) *Managing the 'Unthinkable': policies relating to the sexual abuse of adults with learning disabilities*. London: Family Planning Association.

Brown, H. and Ferns, P. (1991) *Supervising Staff*, video-assisted training pack in the *Bringing People Back Home* series, Bexhill: SETRA.

Brown, H. and Stein, J. (in preparation) *Policies on the Abuse of Vulnerable Adults: a critical review*. Centre for the Applied Psychology of Care, University of Kent.

Brown, H. and Turk, V. (1992) 'Defining sexual abuse as it affects adults with learning difficulties'. *Mental Handicap* 20 (2): 44–55.

Carson, D. (1992) 'Legality of responding to the sexuality of a client with profound learning disabilities'. *Mental Handicap* 20 (2): 85–7.

Craft, A. (1987) 'Mental handicap and sexuality: issues for individuals with a mental handicap, their parents and professionals', in Craft, A. (ed.) *Mental Handicap and Sexuality: Issues and Perspectives*. Tunbridge Wells: Costello.

Craft, A. (1992) *Sex Education for Students with Learning Disabilities: A Guide to Resources*, available from Dr A. Craft, Dept of Learning Disabilities' University of Nottingham Medical School, Queens Medical Centre, Nottingham NG7 2UH.

Craft, A. and Cromby, J. (1991) *Parental Involvement in the Sex Education of Students with Severe Learning Difficulties: A Handbook*, available from Dr A. Craft, Dept of Learning Disabilities, University of Nottingham Medical School, Queens Medical Centre, Nottingham NG7 2UH.

Craft, A. and members of the Nottinghamshire SLD Sex Education Project (1991) *Living Your Life: A Sex Education and Personal Development Programme for Students with Severe Learning Difficulties*. Cambridge: LDA.

Craft, A. and Slack, P. (in press) 'Psychotherapy with a sexually abused client with learning abilities', in Craft, A. and Harris, J. (eds) *Sexual Abuse of Adults with Learning Disabilities*, Kidderminster: British Institute of Learning Disabilities.

Deffenbacher, J. (1985) 'A cognitive-behavioural response and a modest proposal'. *Counselling Psychologist* 13: 261–9.

Dixon, H. (1992) *A Chance to Choose*. Cambridge: LDA.

Dixon, H. and Craft, A. (1992) *Picture Yourself*, four packs of illustrated cards, Cambridge: LDA.

East Sussex County Council (1992) *Sexuality Guidelines*. Brighton: East Sussex County Council.

EMFEC (1991) *Self Advocacy at Work: Training materials for people involved in supporting others to represent themselves*. Further Education and Training Support, Robins Wood House, Robins Wood Road, Nottingham NG8 3NH.

Gunn, M. (1991) *Sex and the Law: A brief guide for staff working with people with learning difficulties*. London: Family Planning Association.

Handy, C. (1976) *Understanding Organisations*. Harmondsworth: Penguin.

Hounslow Social Services Department (1982) *Sexuality of Mentally Handicapped People – Guidelines for Care Staff*. Hounslow Social Services Department.

Hudson, B. (1988) 'Do people with a mental handicap have rights?', *Disability, Handicap and Society* 3 (3): 227–37.

Jackson, S. and Schuler, R. (1985) 'A meta-analysis and conceptual critique of research on role ambiguity and role conflict in work settings', *Organizational Behavior and Human Decision Processes* 31: 16–78.

Jones, J., Kitson, D., Craft, A. and Zadik, T. (1991) 'The sociosexual needs of people with a mental handicap'. *Mental Handicap* 19 (4): 138–42.

Karasek, R. and Theorell, T. (1990) *Healthy Work: Stress, Productivity and the Reconstruction of Working Life*. Basic Books: New York.

Law Commission (1991) *Mentally Incapacitated Adults and Decision Making: An Overview*, Law Commission Consultation Paper No. 119, London: HMSO.

Lewisham Special Needs Sexuality Project (1988) *Sexuality and Special Needs: An introduction to sexuality for people with learning difficulties*, available from Special Needs Sexuality Project, Respite Care Section 340 Lewisham Road, London SE13 6LE.

Mitchell, L. (1985) *Behavioral Intervention in the Sexual Problems of Mentally Handicapped Individuals*. Springfield, Ill.: Charles C. Thomas.

Nottingham Health Authority and Nottinghamshire Social Services Department (1992) *Abuse of Adults with a Mental Handicap/Learning Difficulty: Procedural Guidelines*, available from Dept of Learning Disabilities, University of Nottingham Medical School, Queens Medical Centre, Nottingham NG7 2UH.

Open University (1986) *Patterns for Living*. Milton Keynes: Open University. (Contains a section on personal relationships and sexuality.)

Shelton, D. (1992) 'Client sexual behaviour and staff attitudes: shaping masturbation in an individual with a profound mental and secondary sensory handicap'. *Mental Handicap* 20 (2): 81–4.

Turk, V. and Brown, H. (1992) 'Sexual abuse and adults with learning disabilities'. *Mental Handicap* 20 (2): 56–8.

Walmsley, S. (1989) 'The need for safeguards', in Brown, H. and Craft, A. (eds) *Thinking the Unthinkable: Papers on the Sexual Abuse of People with Learning Difficulties*. London: Family Planning Association.

Watson, G. and Rogers, R. (1980a) 'Sexual instruction for the mildly retarded and normal adolescent: a comparison of educational approaches, parental expectations and pupil knowledge and attitude'. *Health Education Journal* 39 (3): 88–95.

Watson, G. and Rogers, R. (1980b) 'Mildly retarded adolescents – their sexual awareness and education'. *British Journal of Sexual Medicine* June: 38–42.

Whittaker, A. (ed.) (1991) *Supporting Self Advocacy*. London: King's Fund Centre.

2 Working with parents

John Rose and Chris Jones

The lives of people with learning disabilities and the parents with whom they live are inextricably entwined. Pauline Fairbrother, mother to a (then) young woman with a learning disability, writes:

> By the very nature of their handicap they are always overlooked and directed. So not only do mentally handicapped people need sex education and counselling, but so do we, the parents and professionals, the 'overlookers'. Our attitudes must be examined, and if necessary undergo change if mentally handicapped people are ever going to have their sexual needs recognised and met.
>
> (Fairbrother 1983)

The attitudes of parents to sexual and other moral issues are natural, powerful and often positive influences in the lives of their offspring. They cannot be disregarded. Professionals working in the field of learning disabilities cannot hope that they will diminish either with time or by simple counter-argument. They even extend beyond the grave as one middle-aged woman with a learning disability recently confided:

> 'My sadness is that mummy died and she never told me about sex and babies. She just didn't like it. She wouldn't talk about it.'

This chapter examines firstly the different levels at which parents and professionals interact over the sexuality of people with learning disabilities in their care. It is then argued that training for parents around sexual issues is both needed and generally welcomed, but that the concerns and priorities of professionals and parents are very different. A series of workshops exclusively for parents is then described and evaluated.

LEVELS OF INTERACTION

Interaction between parents and professionals can be thought of on four levels:

No interaction
Reacting to incidents
Receiving information
Dialogue: development and education

No interaction

It is common practice for there to be no significant involvement of parents with professionals concerning the sexuality of their offspring. There can be several reasons for this. Either sexuality and learning disability is seen as a non-issue – it just does not exist – or it is seen as the exclusive province of *either* parents *or* professionals.

Sexuality as a non-issue

'What you haven't had, you don't miss. Let sleeping dogs lie, that's what I say.'

There is a strong thread running through the history of people with learning disabilities that portrays them as eternal innocents, blessed with freedom from the curse of sexual feelings (e.g. Craft 1987a). This is consistent with a more general concept of such people being treated as children whatever their chronological age. (This despite the fact that children are far from being asexual.) If sexuality does not exist, there is clearly nothing about which to interact!

This attitude says more about the sexuality of the people holding it, than about those with a learning disability. There is now a rapidly increasing recognition of the human rights of people with learning disabilities (United Nations 1971) and their sexual rights in particular (Harvey 1983; Craft 1987b).

Sexuality as purely a parental concern

'Sex should stay at home where it belongs; it's a family matter.'

It is sometimes held that sex is such a personal matter, and so bound up with the religious and moral values of the family, that no-one outside the family has a right to broach the subject. The privacy of the sexual act itself is mirrored by privacy of talking *about* it, or any related issue.

In truth, sex does not exist in a sealed box in the family home; it is as thoroughly woven into the social fabric of everyday life as the way we eat or do the shopping. To fail to recognise this is itself a powerful attitude about sexuality.

It is a myth that parents generally wish to retain complete control over the education of their children in sexual matters (e.g. Kempton 1975; Kempton and Caparulo 1983). It is a notion often proposed by professionals as a reason to avoid an area of dialogue that *they* find difficult to tackle (Brown 1987). The difficulties of talking about sex, particularly with an older generation of parents, should not be interpreted as a rejection of help with what might be very deep anxieties. Said one mother, widowed in her late seventies, referring to 'it':

'You expect me to talk about it with you, a young man, when even my mother couldn't talk about it with me. And you want to talk about it with my daughter. It's very difficult . . . but it is important, I know that really.'

Another woman and her elderly husband had been written off by Day Care staff, as far as discussion of sexuality was concerned, because they were both staunch Jehovah's Witnesses. It had been assumed that the rigidity of their texts about sexual behaviour made them impervious to outside influence. On the contrary, the parents approached the Day Centre to discuss their son's sexuality. They said that their son needed to be exposed to both factual information about sex and to views other than his own because he had to learn to cope with the real world. Not everyone is a Jehovah's Witness.

Sexuality as purely a professional concern

'I'd much sooner leave it to the experts . . . .'

Another historical thread that has coloured services to people with disabilities is that of the 'medical model'. In essence, the label 'mental handicap' or 'learning disability' consigns the person to a category of human defect that can only be understood, and remedied, by professional expertise. The rapid growth of special resources and training for professionals in the area of formal sex education (e.g. Craft and Members of the Nottinghamshire SLD Sex Education Project 1991, Dixon 1988; Brook Advisory Centres 1987; Kempton

1988) can easily reinforce this belief, with the danger that parental contribution is minimised and devalued. In reality, learning about sexuality is a lifelong and inevitable part of human interaction, not least with one's parents (Kempton 1975). The issue is whether or not this huge area of informal learning is recognised, understood and built upon.

A more recent trend has been deliberately to isolate the adult with a learning disability from the influence of parents. With rare exceptions, parents have no legal rights over the decisions or actions of their adult offspring (Gunn 1991; Robbins 1990). It could be argued that consulting with parents reinforces the myth that the person with a disability is a perpetual child.

David Brandon, editor of the radical journal *Community Living*, writes, somewhat tongue in cheek:

> Recently I spoke to a small branch of the Down's Syndrome Society. It was a bad night for them. I tried ingratiating myself by saying that Britain had some of the most fascist parents in the universe who had single handedly held up the dynamic progress of mental handicap services over the last twenty five years.
>
> (Brandon 1989)

Whilst sympathetic to the aims of the principles of normalisation (Wolfensberger 1972), the strategy of non-involvement of parents does not seem a sensible way of achieving them. The social and private life of a person with a learning disability is often almost entirely controlled by parents or carers (e.g. Lundstrom-Roche 1982), and yet it is exactly this area which is most concerned with real, adult, sexual expression. Attempts at teaching appropriate and adult forms of behaviour, for example, are diminished if more childish expressions are expected in other settings. Talk of forming and valuing sexual relationships is confusing if the idea of such relationships clearly causes anxiety to one's parents. It is more productive to make parental attitudes quite explicit, and then learn to cope with them.

Reacting to incidents

Sexuality as 'a problem'

The first contact between professionals and parents regarding sexuality frequently revolves around an incident of concern to one party or the other. Whilst accepting that some sexual behaviour is clearly inappropriate by the standards of either law or general decency it is often the case that *any* expression of sexuality is seen as a problem.

> A young man and woman with mild learning disabilities were referred to a psychologist attending a Day Centre. The initial problem had been that they were kissing and fondling each other outside the front of the building in breaks and lunchtimes. The Manager had decided that this was unacceptable, and had ordered that they be kept apart. Their behaviour was not decent, and he was worried that it would lead on to 'other things'. The couple could not be separated. They were found in toilets; they were found in store rooms; they were found behind hedges. The young man in particular was becoming aggressive to the staff trying to impose the Manager's ruling. At *this* stage, both sets of parents were contacted because the Manager could not shoulder the risk of an unwanted pregnancy.
>
> (Mitchell 1987)

What had begun as an opportunity for education about sexual behaviour, and a chance to explore with the couple their options for other, more appropriate social contact beyond the Centre, became a conflict of wills with a momentum of its own. Although sharing a problem at this stage with parents might eventually be productive in terms of greater freedom for the couple concerned, it cannot be an ideal way to progress because of the association of sex with anxiety and disapproval on all sides. Indeed, an incident might raise anxiety to such an extent that repressive measures might be taken with long-term consequences:

> A boy in his late teens with a severe learning disability wandered off from a special youth club. He turned up later in the company of a policeman. He had been playing in the streets with some local children, and had been attempting to partly undress a girl aged seven. The boy's father was horrified by the news later that evening when collecting his son from the youth club. Apparently it had occurred before. He decided not to share it with his wife because it would be too upsetting. He took him to the GP who prescribed Androcur to reduce the sexual drive, adding for good measure that: 'sex education for boys like that is the worst thing you can do'. Similar incidents recurred sporadically over the next few years.

When parents are thrown into discussion about sexuality through the emergence of a 'problem' with their son or daughter, it should not be surprising if their attitudes tend towards minimising risk, and consequent reduction of freedom for their offspring. In order to avoid these sensitive and emotional encounters with parents, professional carers may also tend to develop regimes based on minimising sexual expression.

It is clearly in everyone's interests to begin dialogue about sexuality as early as possible in the relationship between professional and parent, and certainly before 'problems' dominate the agenda.

Receiving information

Sexuality as a curricular item

It is now the norm for children with learning difficulties to receive education in sexual matters at school. Indeed it is a legal requirement for the governing body of any Local Authority school either definitely to opt out of sex education, or to 'make, and keep up to date, a separate written statement of their policy with regard to the content and organisation of the relevant part of the curriculum' (Education (No. 2) Act 1986). In fact, the Department of Education and Science strongly encourages and expects *all* schools to develop programmes of 'appropriate and responsible sex education' (DES 1987). In theory, parental involvement in the development of sex education in special schools should be increased by the 1986 Act, both through some being 'parent governors', and by all having the right to attend the statutory annual governors' meeting. In practice, these formal forums are accessible only to the articulate few. This is especially true when discussing sexual matters.

There is a parallel, if slower, growth in the acceptance of educational packages for adults with learning disabilities, usually delivered through colleges of Further Education or Social Services' Day Centres. Parents are often involved only in the sense of being informed in a greater or lesser amount of detail of the package being taught:

> The question of whether to seek parental permission for people's inclusion in the group was considered. It was decided to inform parents at an Open Evening, rather than ask them, as although they might like to know, they had no right over whether or not their adult offspring could attend.
>
> (Marler and Carrol-Williams 1989)

The sense of having no control over whether or how sons and daughters are taught about sexuality can cause parents great anxiety and may lead to confrontation. One mother told of her experience of a local mental handicap hospital:

'The nurse-teacher said that they all have rights, and that he had a directive from the DHSS to say that they should provide sex education. I said 'let me see the directive' and of course he couldn't show me. It's all a great worry.'

Often these anxieties have been addressed by retaining the notion that sex education is something done to people as a package, away from home, and by experts, but by handing over to parents the right to give or withhold consent. Cumbria Social Services Department, for example, produced a 28-page booklet detailing every curricular statement and each one of 85 visual aids used in one of their Adult Training Centres (Cumbria SSD 1983). This was discussed with parents of prospective students, who could either agree or not agree to their participation.

The 'all or none' approach to sex education is fraught with difficulty:

A young woman with Down's Syndrome expressed an interest in joining a course of sex education at her Adult Training Centre. A syllabus was sent to her parents, who duly signed and returned a 'consent slip'. Although she showed initial signs of intense embarrassment at pictures of nakedness and sexual acts, the young student was very interested in the material and learned the factual information well. Long after the end of the course she became increasingly depressed and agitated about many matters, but with a focus on sexuality. The parents blamed 'the course'. Upon investigation they revealed that they had wanted their daughter's participation to learn about sexual matters solely in order to fend off sexual advances and become safe from the risk of sexual exploitation. They had *not* wanted her to understand her feelings as a woman and have sexual desires and aspirations of her own. Their abhorrence was made plain to their daughter.

Clearly the implications of the same written agenda can be understood differently by parent and teacher. Teaching about sexuality is not comparable to teaching someone how to bake a sponge cake; it has to take into account the real lives of the students, which are largely circumscribed by the attitudes of their parents or carers. The occasion of discussing the nature of sex education can be the chance for genuine dialogue, and there is strong evidence to show that the overwhelming majority of parents would welcome this sort of involvement (Goodman, Budner and Lesh 1971; Kempton and Caparulo 1983; Squire 1989). In referring to their experience of addressing large groups of parents about sexuality, Johnson and Kempton (1981) report that:

Over the years, I (Johnson) have been impressed by the response of these parents. There have been hundreds of them now, and they represent something of a cross-section of our society, socio-economically and educationally . . . .

My distinct impression is that professionals have been under-estimating the public. School administrators, teachers, physicians and politicians tend to feel they need to protect the public from the realities of sex.

Dialogue: development and education

Sexuality as an inevitable and valued part of life

'It strikes me that I need education just as much as my daughter.'

To summarise, there is a need to engage professionals and parents and carers in a dialogue about sexuality and learning disability. This would be welcomed by the majority of parents, and would benefit their sons and daughters in many ways. It should take place early in the relationship, and preferably before incidents or problems of a sexual nature dominate the agenda. In part it should relate to the exchange of information, e.g. regarding sex education or legal aspects of sex and learning disabilities, but it is also about discovering, sharing and changing attitudes towards the sexuality of those in their care.

How should this dialogue and education be structured? There are two practical questions to be addressed. Is it best achieved on an individual or on a group basis? Are the needs of parents and professional carers comparable or significantly different?

INDIVIDUAL COUNSELLING OR GROUP WORK?

Individual counselling

Although uncommon it is quite possible for parents to receive on an individual basis both broad and specific help with the sexuality of their offspring:

During the course of a Review meeting at a Day Centre, a mother began to voice concerns about her son's sexual understanding in the light of his prolonged staring at semi-clad bodies of both sexes at the local swimming baths. An appointment was made to meet with a member of staff with a stated interest in this area of work. She talked about the sexual education of her other children and the feeling that it was all closely related to her religious beliefs (Catholic) and a family duty. She was lent *Sex and the Mentally Handicapped – a Guide for Parents and Carers* (Craft and Craft 1982), which she read and found helpful. She returned for two subsequent sessions to discuss her progress with her son's education, aspects of his social behaviour and problems with explaining certain points. The arrangement seemed satisfactory to all concerned, not least to her son.

It is our experience that virtually all parents known to us have concerns about the sexuality of their offspring with a learning disability but these concerns are seldom voiced in the absence of significant 'problems' (see above). It should be good practice to give thought to an individual's sexual needs during regular reviews of progress and planning in other areas of life. This can be included routinely in the system of Individual Programme Planning (e.g. Blunden 1980) now widely adopted in various forms throughout health and social services. It does require commitment and confidence on the part of the professionals running the IPP meeting to raise these issues, and hopefully the skills to do this are being acquired as a result of the growth of training in the area of sexuality (Dixon 1986). Unfortunately, through mutual anxiety about airing the topic, such discussion is often avoided altogether, or dismissed with the statement: 'no problems'.

There are advantages in working with individual parents on sexuality, and sometimes it is the only feasible way of delivering a service (Taylor 1989). The counselling can be tailored exactly to meet perceived needs, and the practicalities of where, when and how the work is done are often easier to arrange. There are, however, other advantages in working with larger numbers of people.

Group work

There are several reasons for working with *groups* of parents and carers on issues concerned with sexuality, most of which are common to *any* work with parents (e.g. Cunningham and Davis 1985; McConkey 1985).

Economy

The larger the group, the more economical it becomes in terms of parents reached per hour of professional time. However, beyond a certain size, there is a cost in terms of what is being achieved between group members, and this is a critical decision to be made when setting it up.

Mutual support

It is often reported by parents that they listen well to other parents because they 'know what it's like'. It is very reassuring to find that other parents have had exactly the same kind of worries and doubts as oneself. There is also pressure from peers in a group which is quite absent in individual counselling. In facilitating a group of parents, points are often most powerfully made by reinforcing something pertinent said by a certain parent, rather than by presenting the same thing cold as yet another professional fact.

Motivation

Parents often feel very committed to attend a group because of a sense of loyalty to the other members. This is particularly the case when the group is fairly small. Also there is no doubt that it can be made into an enjoyable social occasion, with a sense of having participated in something that was fun to do.

Reduced pressure

The work of a group does not exclusively focus on an individual or individual problem. This is especially important in the area of sexuality, where exposure of personal feelings can be very threatening. Much of the material dealt with is on a broader canvas, control over whether or not to reveal personal issues being left with the individual.

Creative solutions

Several people working on a particular problem are more likely than an individual to throw up a variety of ideas about it. Professional facilitators of groups are as likely to gain insights into issues surrounding sexuality as are the parental participants.

Ongoing support

Sometimes workshops specific to sexuality are grafted onto a programme of parents' meetings which happen regularly anyway. This can be an advantage because sexuality is less likely to be seen as pathological or as a problem area if it is one of a series of other topics. Equally it can be envisaged that the success of parents' groups especially established to deal with sexual issues might continue as a mutual support group with a wider brief.

THE NEEDS OF PARENTS V. THE NEEDS OF PROFESSIONALS

Whilst the parents of people with learning disabilities and those that care for them professionally both need guidance and training regarding sexuality, it is by no means clear that both groups need the same sort of help. Indeed there are important differences to take into account.

The focus

'I'll tell you why you find this group of parents difficult. You see, we only have our own son or daughter to think about, and my word we know them well. But we don't have the interest in the others that you do. It's very different for you.'

A parent comes to group with a lifelong responsibility for (usually) one person – their own son or daughter. That is not to say that there is no sympathy or understanding of other people's situations, but it is not their direct concern. The professional carer, however, may be responsible for a hundred or more individuals with learning disabilities depending on the job. These are very different perspectives.

Priorities

'When we took our daughter for short-term care we were always asked: 'Is she on the pill? You really should consider it'. When I asked why, they said our daughter had a right to make sexual relationships. I said they should keep a better eye on the young men there! I said they should supervise the girls better!'

Surveys of parental attitudes to the sexuality of their offspring are fairly consistent, albeit small scale (Goodman, Budner and Lesh, 1971; Fischer and Krajicek 1974; Kempton 1979; Squire 1989). Generally they concern anxieties about the risk of being molested or exploited, and daughters becoming pregnant, about getting into trouble with the law (especially males) and about frustration at not being able to achieve full sexual roles.

Attitude surveys with professionals have shown a gradual change over the last twenty years. A range of professional groups have demonstrated a greater willingness to acknowledge and assist with the development of the sexuality of people with learning disabilities in recent years (Rose and Holmes 1991). Professional concerns are now more likely to revolve around approval for risk-taking, usually in the context of helping people in their care engage in age-appropriate, integrated social activities. They are often more concerned with the legal framework in which they operate, and with the area of human rights of people with learning disabilities. They are interested in factual information about the sexual development of people with disabilities, and about issues of policy-making by whatever authority they work for.

These are the areas primarily addressed by training packages for professional people both in areas of general sexuality (Heather 1984) and specifically in relation to learning disabilities (Brock 1990, Dixon 1986).

There are instances of training in sexuality for mixed groups of parents and professionals (e.g. Brantlinger 1983; Stevens *et al.* 1988), but in general, professional involvement is as a leader, not as a co-participant. Their personal priorities really are very different, and frustration at this difference in perception is often a key area that parents wish to air between themselves.

Timescale

'People come and go. We see a different social worker every six months. But who's left holding the baby? That's what I want to know.'

Parents generally feel a deep and lifelong commitment to the wellbeing of their sons and daughters. They usually try to secure and approve a lifestyle for them to last beyond their own death. These natural tendencies are especially marked when dealing with offspring who are perceived as unable to fend for themselves. The timescale for parents is very long indeed, and if they are pessimistic about change, they often have good reasons for this.

Not only do professionals often have many clients under their care at any one time, but through career changes, they have often had experiences of very many more, the destinies of whom are now unknown. It should not be surprising if conflict sometimes arises between the short-term visions of a professional and the longer-term realism of a parent. These issues are expertly reviewed elsewhere by Hilary Brown (1987).

Consideration of the range of interactions between parents and professionals, and the perceived needs of parents for dialogue and education led the authors to consider running a series of groups exclusively for parents, the first of which began in January 1988.

ASSEMBLING THE GROUPS: OUR EXPERIENCES

The formation of parents' groups can be a challenge. There are many reasons why parents may be reluctant to attend groups and work-shops (McConkey 1985). These include experiences of 'help' from professionals and groups in the past which they found impossible to reconcile with their own views or irrelevant to their own needs. This may be particularly important with an emotive topic such as sexuality. Parents of adults will generally have been caring for their offspring for many years and may feel there is little more they can do or learn to help their offspring develop. There may also be many practical reasons why parents do not attend workshops: they are often busy people, they may also need someone to care for their child while they attend.

However, this work was initiated after a request by parents, through a local MENCAP group, expressing a desire to learn more about sex education for their sons and daughters. After circulating a letter to a large number of parents a group of eleven expressed an interest in attending a series of four sessions.

The parents were then consulted by letter as to convenient times for the group sessions. Considerable advance notice was given of the time and dates for each session. Unfortunately as the parents came from a wide geographical area it meant that some parents had to travel a long distance. The parents who attended this group were committed because of a particular interest in sexuality. This no doubt contributed to its success (Rose 1990). However, because of the importance of opening a dialogue about sexuality we felt that it was necessary to try and develop this work with other parents.

We then started to focus attention on parents whose offspring were attending either Colleges of Further Education or Adult Training Centres. Here we made initial contact through the management and teaching staff.

Various methods were used to bring parents together. These have included a written notice to all parents explaining the ideas behind the workshops and a rationale for them. Where possible these were then followed up by personal contact either by telephone or in person. Great efforts were made to do this especially if it was felt the parents' attendance was particularly important, e.g. their son or daughter was about to start a programme of sex education. This was then often followed by an initial group meeting to introduce some of the issues around sexuality. For successful groups it was often necessary to send out several letters and use telephone calls as 'reminders'. On one occasion our attempts to start a group were unsuccessful with only three parents attending on the first evening. This may have been due to several reasons. Personal contact and reminders had not been used. Also, there had been no contact with the group by the college for several months and we later discovered by personal contact that some parents had found previous meetings of the same forum to be unhelpful.

Workshops were held at different times of day depending on the needs of the group of parents. For evening groups it was sometimes necessary to provide care for sons and daughters. This was done by either holding the session to coincide with a social activity or club which some could attend or for a member of college or training centre staff to provide a leisure activity for them at a different location at the same site as the parents' meeting.

With persistence it has been possible to develop a number of groups for parents. However, our experience has taught us that flexibility is an important factor in their success.

DIFFERENCES BETWEEN GROUPS OF PARENTS: THE IMPORTANCE OF A FLEXIBLE APPROACH

Like the rest of society, parents of people with learning disabilities are a heterogeneous group. There are many differences between parents which need to be recognised and respected. From our experience of working with parents we have found differences not only between individuals but also between groups.

Major changes have occurred in attitudes towards sexuality over recent years. In general, older parents tend to be more cautious in their attitudes towards sexuality which is much more likely to have been a taboo subject in their youth. Services to people with learning disabilities and expectations for them have changed dramatically in some areas in a relatively short time (e.g. Allen, Pahl and Quine 1990). Hence older parents will have different experiences of care, often spending years protecting their offspring from the community and entry into institutions. However, this is not to say that parents cannot adapt to changes. In a recent workshop an elderly mother of a woman with Down's syndrome commented:

'I sometimes wonder if we've been overprotective. When our daughter went on holiday with the centre she went rock climbing and abseiling. She had a great time. We would never have thought of letting her do that. It must be good for her.'

Younger parents may expect their son or daughter to take a much more active part in community life. Differences between individual offspring will also have a major effect on how parents perceive sexuality as an issue for them and their son or daughter (Chapman and Pitceathly 1985). The extent to which individuals develop and take an interest in sexual matters is clearly variable (Monat 1982). The degree of offspring's learning disability will also influence how a parent perceives sexuality as an issue. One parent commented:

'I'm not sure if this (sexuality) applies to my son as he's profoundly handicapped.'

He later confided that his son masturbated frequently, often in public. It is sometimes much easier for both parents and professionals to deny the sexual needs of people with more severe handicaps. Needs are usually just as great although they may need to be considered differently.

Parents with a specific interest in the sexuality of their offspring, such as those with whom we worked initially, may also be prepared to discuss things more fully and openly at an earlier stage than other groups. They may have considered the topic more carefully before and have more to bring to a group from their own experience.

As indicated earlier, differences in religious belief will have an important influence on attitudes to sexuality which also needs to be considered. Differences of this kind need to be taken into account when considering group work with parents on the topic of sexuality. Some general characteristics of a group can be anticipated from the way a group is selected: Have they expressed a special interest? How old are they? Are there any predominant religious beliefs? What are their offspring like? Different methods of selection will tend to 'cluster' parents with particular characteristics, e.g. parents whose offspring attend Adult Training Centres will generally be older than those who attend school or college. With such a large number of variables it soon became apparent that each group required an approach tailored to its individual characteristics.

This was especially important as the aim of the workshops was not for professionals to teach and preach to parents. Rather it was to help parents consider issues and concerns and talk with other parents in an open way, so that hopefully they would become more confident in coping with sexual issues. It was felt essential to try and meet the group where they were and develop the workshop around them, rather than slavishly to follow a set of procedures.

In general group sessions lasted one and a half to two hours and were arranged fortnightly but with some flexibility depending on participants' requirements. Groups were generally restricted to parents only. Workshops to date have consisted of between four and six sessions, but there is clearly scope for extending them.

We have not yet offered more intense workshops, e.g. one day or two day workshops, as participants have found short sessions to be convenient. This may be considered in the future.

WORKSHOP CONTENT

Even though it was felt essential for parents to feel comfortable with discussion in the group and have a large say in the format of the workshop we also felt that it was necessary to provide a structure which would use the relatively short time available efficiently.

In general, the first or introductory session contained a number of exercises which set the scene yet invited participation at any level. It was also used to introduce group members to each other and assist with the planning of future sessions.

The initial session

Sessions generally started with brief personal introductions by the workshop facilitators, then went on to introduce group members.

The amount of time required to introduce group members depended on the previous experience of the group in working together. If the group was largely unfamiliar with each other, participants would be asked to pair up with someone they did not know, and exchange names and information about themselves and their offspring. Then they had to report back to the group about the person they had just been talking to, thus giving everyone a contact in the group and an early opportunity to speak both to someone else and in the group. Alternatively, if the group members knew each other, a useful method of introduction was to ask participants to say their names and 'something about their son or daughter'. This would often provide a useful insight into the group and their needs.

During the first session, the rules of the group were always made clear. It was expected that discussion within the group would remain *confidential* to that group. Also that everyone should feel free to express their views and that *all opinions are valid*.

The workshop facilitators also made it clear that the sessions were not intended to find 'answers' but to provide a forum for group discussion and exploration of attitudes and feelings. Some factual material would be presented and hopefully integrating this would make future decisions easier and better informed, but clearly this could not be guaranteed.

After introductions the first activity would often take the form of an illustrated talk, using case studies where the sexual aspects of the lives of people with learning disabilities either had been allowed to develop, or had been restricted or misunderstood. This provided examples of how sexuality could play an important part in the lives of people with learning disabilities in many different ways. It gave some parents the opportunity to relate the material to their own offspring and make potentially difficult revelations. For example, when discussing a man with a learning disability who was attracted to younger boys, one parent was quick to comment:

> We had this problem with our (son). While at school he would often seek out the younger boys to play with. We were very worried. Now he's at college we think it's stopped.

Using other examples gave parents the chance to express their fears and set an agenda.

> 'It's not my daughter I'm worried about, it's the rest of the world.'

> 'You get lots of hostility. I've had year after year of hitting my head against a brick wall, society doesn't understand.'

> 'When us parents go, that's the worry.'

Some examples included references to sex education. Parents were always interested in this aspect of the discussion and often keen to be involved in any programme. In some instances where education had already been done there was sometimes considerable suspicion and antagonism:

> 'These people (staff) ought to think of the damage they can do to the child emotionally.'

> 'We had no problem with (son's name) until they started up this sex education business. *Then* we had terrible trouble with him (unspecified). He settled down again though, but we don't think it's a good thing at all.'

Reflecting on the lives of other people often made parents consider their relationship with their offspring in a different way, as one elderly mother commented:

'It's not easy, but I think we should let our (daughter's name) have more independence.'

Specific areas of interest were generally very clear from the first session, and these were taken into account in planning the rest of the workshop.

Subsequent sessions

Here we will simply present the range of techniques we used which could be used in any combination depending on the needs of the group.

Quizzes

During the workshops we made extensive use of the quizzes described by Dixon (1986). All of these questionnaires were useful as a means of imparting knowledge and promoting discussion in a non-threatening way. Participants were asked to fill in the questionnaires by themselves but it was made clear that it was not a test of their knowledge and that we did not want to see individual answers. They were then asked to discuss the answers in pairs or small groups before a more general discussion in the main group.

The quiz we used most frequently was 'Sex and Mental Handicap' which most parents found informative and useful. However, some questions which related to Down's syndrome were identified to be only of 'academic interest' by one parent whose child did not have the syndrome.

The quiz 'Sex and the Law' was also of interest to many parents. However, this was generally used in a shortened form concentrating on the most relevant questions to the group. Again, it was generally received positively, but there was sometimes considerable surprise about the legal independence of people with a learning disability over the age of eighteen. It also raised the issue of rights:

'It's all very well talking about the rights of our children, but parents have rights too you know!'

'We hear a lot about people's rights these days but not much about responsibilities.'

The final quiz, 'Aspects of Sexuality', was used less frequently and only with groups of parents who appeared to have considered many of the issues and were generally willing to accept their offspring's sexuality.

The experience of handicap and sexuality

Other activities attempted to bridge the gap between the sexual experiences and opportunities of people with and without learning disabilities. One way of doing this was to ask the group members to say how they had learnt about various sexual topics, e.g. 'how a baby is made'. These were listed on a piece of paper or white board. They were then asked to list how their sons and daughters may have found out about the same topics. These were also listed and compared. This activity gave insight into a number of issues, including differences due to handicap and generation; also the inevitability that people would learn something (correct or incorrect) and the importance of clear information and teaching.

Another activity which examined issues of handicap used case studies. Parents were split into small groups and asked to discuss case studies which illustrated aspects of parent–child relationships. The studies focused on one aspect of sexuality, e.g. masturbation, pregnancy, abortion and homosexuality. The first cases related to families whose children did not have learning disabilities and a second set examined similar issues where a child had a learning disability. Parents then fed back to the large group where attitudes to the different situations were discussed.

Comparing situations in this way provided a graphic illustration of how perception of a learning disability could change parental behaviour. It also demonstrated to parents that their children were adults with adult feelings and needs which presented challenges to them.

Examining personal attitudes

Another exercise allowed the examination of individual attitudes. This used two sets of cards, one with statements relating to sexuality in general, e.g. 'People should not be told about sexual matters until they ask about them', and the other set relating to people with learning disabilities, e.g. 'People with learning disabilities should not be told about sexual matters until they ask about them'. Parents were asked to take at least one card from each set which was placed face down. They were then asked to place the card on a continuum from 'agree' to 'disagree' (defined as a line down the middle of the room) and then give their reasons for placing the card in their selected position.

No debate was allowed until everyone had placed their cards. When all of the cards had been placed people were given the opportunity to move cards and state their reasons why. This process usually gave rise to much lively discussion. Many favourable comments were made about this exercise including:

'Made me really think about what I believed and why.'

'It is really interesting to hear everyone's views and how they are different.'

'Later, when I got home and thought about the cards, I thought about other possible views.'

Video presentation

Another useful way of stimulating discussion was the use of the video *Baby First* (Yorkshire TV 1984). This includes a film recorded in the USA of a couple with learning disabilities who are married and have a child. The couple were receiving a considerable amount of support. Even though parents were quick to comment that there was much that we were not told about them and that they were 'obviously much less handicapped than our (offspring)', the couple in the video generally received approval from the parent's group for their right to marry and have children. In a debate about the appropriateness of the state paying for a full-time nurse to help the parents, one group member was quick to defend this right:

'Of course they (the state) should pay to help support them (parents with learning disabilities) to bring up a child. They don't think twice about paying for a heart transplant or other expensive operations. I think that child deserves as much chance in life as any other.'

A possible framework for action

Some emphasis was placed on activities that helped participants explore ways of thinking about the way they reacted to their own sons and daughters.

One way in which this was done was to set the scene giving a brief presentation detailing possible 'levels of response' in terms of three broad categories:

Restriction/Punishment

Actively denying opportunities, e.g. segregation by sex, punishment for displaying sexual behaviour.

Tolerance/Acceptance

Accepting some sexual behaviour, e.g. masturbation, but not teaching people about their bodies. Reacting if necessary and acknowledging sexuality but little more.

Nurture/Development

Behaving proactively by helping to educate. Also responding to sexuality in a positive way, viewing sexual and other behaviour as opportunities for personal development.

It was often possible to refer to these categories as a framework in other discussions and activities.

Problem solving

Another method which was described and practised was problem solving (Dixon, 1986; D'Zurilla and Goldfried, 1971). This was presented as a method of analysis that could be used by them to appraise and get the best out of situations which they may find themselves in.

How to talk more effectively with your son or daughter

This was an exercise adapted from 'Counselling Role Plays' (Dixon 1986). It consisted of an introduction presenting the parent as a helper who could use a range of counselling skills to assist their offspring. The group was then split into threes with one parent playing the role of the parent, another the child and the other observing the techniques used. They were then given roles and support from facilitators if requested. Many parents found this difficult, particularly role playing a person with a learning disability. One participant commented:

'I keep thinking about what my (daughter) would do. The role doesn't seem quite right'

However, it was generally seen as a useful exercise by most parents.

'It's shown me that I should learn to listen and ask a few more questions rather than come to immediate conclusions.'

'It was interesting to see different approaches.'

Sex education

Sex education was always given some time as a topic. Many parents wanted to know more about it as a general topic but also to find out more about what their offspring would be or had been receiving. Where possible the people who were responsible for teaching their sons and daughters were invited to give a presentation or be prepared to answer questions. Education was introduced at a later stage in the workshops and by this time participants generally saw some value in the teaching and were able to enter into serious debate, even if not entirely agreeing with the prospect of sex education for their own son or daughter. However, it was always emphasised that it was important to find out what their children knew, meet them where they were and to realistic about their needs.

'Explaining it like that it doesn't seem such a bad idea after all.'

'I still can't see the point of it for my (son). He doesn't really understand. But it is important.'

Time was usually made available for the parents to express concerns. Sometimes this was quite difficult and had to be dealt with sensitively. Often simply airing these in a group of other parents seemed to help and would engage support and help from other members of the group. It also provided an opportunity for the group facilitators to help.

Other information

Finally, giving information about where to go for further assistance was seen as an important function of the workshops. These included both local support services, e.g. CTLOs, and national agencies, for example SPOD, FPA and Brook Advisory Centres. Some information was also given on useful reading material such as Craft and Craft (1982); Forshaw *et al.* (1988); Shepherd School Sex Education Monitoring Group (1991).

EVALUATION

Various methods of evaluation were used to assess the effectiveness of the workshops. These included verbal feedback at the end of each session and workshop; also a written feedback form requesting comments, both positive and negative. Finally, an attempt was made to use an adapted version of Brantlinger's (1987) attitude inventory.

Participants were requested to complete a copy of the inventory both before and after the workshop. The reasons for using the inventory were carefully explained and the anonymity of individual replies emphasised. Some participants were interested in the question-naire and were keen to discuss it further. However, the inventory clearly distressed a significant minority of parents, some of whom refused to fill it in. One parent who had previously said she would attend refused to come to a series of workshops after receiving it. Others were unable to answer large numbers of questions, or said they found it 'unnecessary' and difficult to complete. Previous research (Dupras and Tremblay, 1976; Chapman and Pitceathly, 1985; Squire, 1989) suggests that people with deep feelings of disapproval to programmes of sex education are reluctant to fill in questionnaires about issues of sexuality. As such it is likely that the questionnaire was seen as threatening by some parents. The questionnaire seemed to be deterring the parents that we wanted to attend most, so we stopped using it after the second group. As there was a considerable amount of missing data from these groups we are unable to report any results. What became clear is that we need to examine other methods of evaluation for these groups.

We were able to collect a large number of comments, both written and verbal. In general, comments were favourable:

'All of these meetings were very good and I'm glad I was able to come to them all.'

'(The workshop) should be compulsory for all parents.'

'When is the next? I'm looking forward to more of these.'

Other comments revealed that they had found the discussion supportive and useful:

'Discussion was easier than I thought.'

'Interesting to hear other people's attitudes.'

Comments on the specific activities varied between the different groups. The activities examining attitudes were generally well received:

'To me the best evening, not only factual but made me really think about what I believed and why.'

'This was a great evening, it gave me a chance to see things in a different way and change my mind if needs be.'

Many parents reported being reassured about the education their sons and daughters were receiving or were about to receive:

'Helpful to know what our kids are being taught and how.'

'Reassuring to know how the education is carried out.'

However some parents expressed concerns:

'I'd like to see some more of those materials and be kept right up to date on progress, so that I know exactly what stage things are.'

'I'm still concerned that the teaching should be done in a Christian moral framework.'

There were some criticisms of the workshops. These were generally about the time available for discussion (often too little). Some parents also made it clear that they found it difficult to relate some of the material to their own offspring, and with a wide range of abilities represented in each group this was perhaps understandable. However, most parents saw this difficulty and we tried to make the workshops relevant to the needs of individuals without being threatening.

CONCLUSION

We believe it is essential to have a dialogue between parents and professionals about the sexuality of people with learning disabilities. This dialogue can take place in many different settings and will vary depending on individual circumstances.

From our experience parents are interested in the sexuality of their offspring but it is important that parents and professionals meet as equals and respect each other's views. One way of doing this is in the form of a workshop designed to meet the needs and interests of groups of parents. Evaluation of these workshops suggests that parents have found them interesting and useful.

We too have learnt a considerable amount by listening carefully to the parents who attended the workshops. Without doubt our own professional work in this area is now tempered with both a greater realism and respect for the views of the parents to whom we relate.

ACKNOWLEDGEMENTS

Thanks are due to the parents who attended the workshops for their participation and ideas. Also to the professionals who helped with the organisation of the groups and contributed to some of the sessions.

REFERENCES

Allen, P., Pahl, J. and Quine, L. (1990) *Care Staff in Transition: The Impact on Staff of the Changing Services for People with Mental Handicap*. London: HMSO.

Baby First (1984), video with Dr Miriam Stoppard, available from Yorkshire TV, Leeds, UK.

Blunden, R. (1980) *Individual Plans for Mentally Handicapped People: A Draft Procedural Guide*. Cardiff: Mental Handicap in Wales Applied Research Unit.

Brandon, D. (1989) 'We can talk but can we dance to their tune?' (Editorial), *Community Living* 2 (2): 2–3.

Brantlinger, E. (1983) 'Measuring variation and change of attitudes of residential care staff toward the sexuality of mentally retarded persons'. *Mental Retardation* 21: 17–23.

Brantlinger, E. (1987) 'Influencing staff attitudes', in Craft, A. (ed.) *Mental Handicap and Sexuality: Issues and Perspectives*. Tunbridge Wells: Costello.

Brock, E. (1990) *Sex Matters: Issues of Sexuality and Sex Education*. Hove: Pavilion Publishing.

Brook Advisory Centres (1987) *Not a Child Anymore* (teaching package), Birmingham: Brook Advisory Centres.

Brown, H. (1987) 'Working with parents', in Craft, A. (ed.). *Mental Handicap and Sexuality: Issues and Perspectives*. Tunbridge Wells: Costello.

Chapman, J.W. and Pitceathly, A.S. (1985) 'Sexuality and mentally handicapped people: issues of sex education, marriage, parenthood, and care staff attitudes'. *Australian and New Zealand Journal of Developmental Disabilities* 10 (4): 227–35.

Craft, A. (1987a) 'Mental handicap and sexuality: issues for individuals with a mental handicap, their parents and professionals'. in Craft, A. (ed.) *Mental Handicap and Sexuality: Issues and Perspectives*. Tunbridge Wells: Costello.

Craft, A. (1987b) *Mental Handicap and Sexuality: Issues and Perspectives*. Tunbridge Wells: Costello.

Craft, A. and Members of the Nottinghamshire SLD Sex Education Project (1991) *Living Your Life: A Sex Education and Personal Development Programme for Students with Severe Learning Difficulties*. Cambridge: LDA.

Craft, M. and Craft, A. (1982) *Sex and the Mentally Handicapped: A Guide for Parents and Carers* (revised edn). London and New York: Routledge & Kegan Paul.

Cumbria Social Services Department (1983) *Health and Sex Education Programme*. Mill Lane ATC: Cumbria SSD.

Cunningham, C. and Davis, H. (1985) *Working with Parents: A Framework for Collaboration*. Milton Keynes: Open University Press.

Department of Education and Science (1987) *Sex Education at School*, Circular No. 11/87, London: DES.

Dixon, H. (1986) *Options for Change: A Staff Training Handbook on Personal Relationships and Sexuality for People with a Mental Handicap*. London: Family Planning Association/BIMH.

Dixon, H. (1988) *Sexuality and Mental Handicap: An Educator's Resource Book*. Cambridge: LDA.

Dupras, A. and Tremblay, R. (1976) 'Path analysis of parents' conservatism towards sex education of their mentally handicapped children'. *American Journal of Mental Deficiency* 81 (2): 162–8.

D'Zurilla, T.J. and Goldfried, M.R. (1971) 'Problem solving and behavior modification'. *Journal of Abnormal Psychology* 78: 107–26.

Education (No. 2) Act (1986), London: HMSO.

Fairbrother, P. (1983) 'The parents' viewpoint', in Craft, A. and Craft, M. (eds) *Sex Education and Counselling for Mentally Handicapped People*. Tunbridge Wells: Costello.

Fischer, H.E. and Krajicek, M.J. (1974) 'Sexual development of the moderately retarded child: level of information and parental attitudes'. *Mental Retardation* 12 (3): 28–32.

Forshaw, I., Keate, W.R.B., Newnham, C. and Stevens, S. (1988) *Right to Know? Information about Sex Education for Parents*, available from Dr S. Stevens, Bell House, Rectory Lane, London SW17 9PS.

Goodman, L., Budner, S. and Lesh, B. (1971) 'The parents' role in sex education for the retarded'. *Mental Retardation* 9 (1): 43–5.

Gunn, M.J. (1991) *Sex and the Law: A brief Guide for Staff Working with People with Learning Difficulties*. London: Family Planning Association.

Harvey, R. S. (1983) 'The sexual rights of mentally handicapped people'. *Mental Handicap* 11 (3): 123–5.

Heather, B. (1984) *Sharing: A Handbook for those Involved in Training in Personal Relationships and Sexuality*. London: Family Planning Association.

Johnson, W. and Kempton, W. (1981) *Sex Education and Counseling for Special Groups*. Springfield, Ill.: Charles C. Thomas.

Kempton, W. (1975) 'Sex education: a co-operative effort between parent and teacher'. *Exceptional Children* May: 531–5.

Kempton, W. (1979) *Sex Education for Persons with Disabilities that Hinder Learning: A Teacher's Guide*. Pennsylvania: Planned Parenthood of SE Pennsylvania.

Kempton, W. (1988) *Life Horizons 1: The Physiological and Emotional Aspects of Being Male and Female*. Five slide programmes (over 500 slides). *Life Horizons 2: The Moral, Social and Legal Aspects of Sexuality*. Seven slide programmes (over 600 slides), Santa Monica, Calif.: Stanfield Film Assoc. Available from Concord Video and Film Council, 201 Felixstowe Rd, Ipswich IP3 9BJ.

Kempton, W. and Caparulo, F. (1983) 'Counselling parents and care staff on the needs of mentally handicapped people', in Craft, A. and Craft, M. (eds) *Sex Education and Counselling for Mentally Handicapped People*. Tunbridge Wells: Costello.

Lundstrom-Roche, F. (1982) 'Sex roles and mentally handicapped people'. *Mental Handicap* 10 (1): 29–30.

McConkey, R. (1985) *Working with Parents: A Practical Guide for Teachers and Therapists*. London: Croom-Helm.

Marler, R. and Carrol-Williams, B. (1989) 'Groupwork on life events and sexuality with adults living in a mental handicap hospital'. *Mental Handicap* 17: 119–22.

Mitchell, L.K. (1987) 'Intervention in the inappropriate sexual behaviour of individuals with mental handicaps', in Craft, A. (ed.) *Mental Handicap and Sexuality: Issues and Perspectives*. Tunbridge Wells: Costello.

Monat, R.K. (1982) *Sexuality and the Mentally Handicapped*. San Diego: College Hill Press.

Robbins, B. (1990) *Ordinary Love. The Sexuality of People with Learning Difficulties*. Bristol: University of Bristol.

Rose, J. (1990) 'Accepting and developing the sexuality of people with mental handicaps: working with parents'. *Mental Handicap* 18 (1): 4–6.

Rose, J. and Holmes, S. (1991) 'An evaluation of the effectiveness of workshops in changing staff attitudes to the sexuality of people with a mental handicap: a comparison of one and three-day workshops'. *Mental Handicap Research* 4 (1): 67–79.

Shepherd School Sex Education Monitoring Group (1991) *Now They're Growing Up* . . . . Series of booklets for parents, available from Shepherd School, Harvey Rd, Nottingham NG8 3BB.

Squire, J. (1989) 'Sex education for pupils with severe learning difficulties: a survey of parent and staff attitudes'. *Mental Handicap* 17: 66–9.

Stevens, S., Evered, C., O'Brien, T. and Wallace, E. (1988) 'Sex education: who needs it?' *Mental Handicap* 16 (4): 166–70.

Taylor, O. (1989) 'Teaching parents about their impaired adolescents' sexuality'. *American Journal of Maternal Child Nursing* 14: 109–12.

United Nations (1971) *Declaration of General and Special Rights of the Mentally Handicapped*. New York: UN Dept of Social Affairs.

Wolfensberger, W. (1972) *The Principles of Normalisation in Human Services*. Toronto: NIMR.

3 Understanding and responding to difficult sexual behaviour

Hilary Brown and Sheila Barrett

INTRODUCTION

Sexual behaviour is a significant cause of the admission and readmission of people with learning disabilities to hospital (see Campbell *et al*. 1982). In order to fulfil the commitment to provide an ordinary life to all people with learning disabilities it is essential that we work towards some understanding of its roots and begin to acquire the expertise to intervene and to manage difficult sexual behaviour in community settings. In this chapter we want to explore how sexual behaviour is learned, how difficult sexual behaviour develops and to suggest a coherent model of intervention in terms of management and treatment, thereby outlining the competencies which services need to develop. The chapter shows how staff groups can work proactively with the small minority of people with learning disabilities whose sexual behaviour has damaging consequences for them or impinges unacceptably on others. It also highlights the responsibility of managers to support staff with appropriate supervision, structures and resources. This requires an overview of:

— the issues relating to sexuality and people with learning disabilities
— current practice in responding to challenging behaviour
— the generic literature on sexual development and pathology.

For a literature review specifically on sexual offenders with learning disabilities see Breen and Turk (in preparation).

Whereas staff feel clear in the face of self-injury or aggression to others, intervening to redirect or reshape an individual's sexual behaviour raises many difficult issues and dilemmas. For example, how would a member of staff weigh up the possibility of replacing sexual behaviour which has been directed at women colleagues with pornographic magazines or videos? How should members of staff sensitively intervene to stop someone masturbating in a public place without inducing feelings of shame or humiliation? Thus, while the processes advocated here will echo the recent literature on challenging behaviours we would argue that there are some special issues at stake and some particular skills which are needed to address them in an ethical and responsible way. It is difficult to persuade staff to be objective and thoughtful about violence or self-injury, but even more so to ask them to suspend judgement in an area which, in many cultural and religious frameworks, is so powerfully tied in to notions of good and evil. When we assert that sexual behaviour is a reflection of what we have learned rather than of who we are, we are disturbing some very powerful beliefs. Viewed from this perspective the deprivation and distortion of service users' sexual behaviour exposes the abnormal sexual climate which exists, both overtly and covertly, in many services.

The chapter begins by setting some boundaries around what constitutes difficult sexual behaviour, explores the possible origins of difficult sexual behaviour and the way it may be being maintained in current environments and suggests strategies for initial screening and assessment. We then go on to a discussion of intervention strategies. Lastly, we examine the systems and structures which need to be in place in organizations which serve people with challenging sexual behaviours to help them maintain positive approaches and contain the inevitable anxiety which such behaviour occasions.

DEFINITIONS

When we come to decide how we need to act in the face of difficult sexual behaviour we are immediately faced with a series of dilemmas. Which behaviours do we categorise as sexual? Which of these are in the person's control? What is difficult and for whom? Is there any agreement about what healthy sexuality might look like? Are some behaviours considered a 'problem' because the person has a learning disability where they would be deemed perfectly normal for non-handicapped persons? The processes whereby sexual behaviours come to be perceived as a problem are by no means straightforward. A minority may have been 'defined' through the courts, while others will present problems to care-givers or family members. Some individuals will have well-documented histories which follow them wherever they go, while others are followed by rumour or innuendo.

The first step is to put some boundaries around the behaviours which we are considering. Legal definitions stress the importance of consent, with non-consensual sexual intercourse or behaviour constituting rape or indecent assault. The law also prohibits certain partners, notably specific relatives (i.e. incest), children under sixteen or, for homosexual relationships, young men under twenty-one and certain acts (such as anal intercourse or homosexual acts in public). Within services there is anxiety that people may break the law but usually difficult behaviour is contained, because those responsible act on the basis that people with learning disabilities offend unwittingly and may not be clear about social or sexual boundaries.

We will explore how this 'containment' can be achieved and suggest an approach which does not minimise the complexity of the problems which are faced by staff and carers nor dull the knife-edge on which services perch, in terms of their management of risk. The behaviours which cause concern range from inappropriate masturbation and sexual harassment of other service users or staff, to serious assault or exploitation. They may be problematical because they are repeated frequently or, if sporadic, loom large in the awareness of staff on account of the potential threat they represent. They inevitably confront staff with complicated decisions and management strategies.

WHAT IS 'DIFFICULT'?

As a starting point it is important to refine our ideas about what creates difficulties and make some judgements about when it is appropriate for services to intervene. People with learning disabilities are often restricted in their sexual options by the prejudices and anxieties of their carers, staff or the general public. The misrepresentation of people with learning disabilities as innocent and childlike is as damaging to them as the more blatant charge of being 'oversexed' and menacing which fed the eugenics movement at the beginning of this century. These powerful stereotypes, even when they are hidden beneath more enlightened dogma, lead to people's sexual behaviour being differentially judged against idealized standards or unconscious fears. We therefore specifically exclude from the category of difficult sexual behaviours, those behaviours which would be considered normal or acceptable in a non-handicapped person of the same age. Knowledge of normal sexual development and of the physiology of sexual arousal will help to ensure that people with learning disabilities are not inappropriately scapegoated for being sexual *per se*. In the past privileges were withdrawn from people in hospital because they had had wet dreams, or they were taunted on account of having an erection, both being involuntary reflexes. This is not to say that these episodes do not sometimes cause difficulties or embarrassment for the people around that individual but that the problem is theirs and should be dealt with as such. Later in the chapter we provide some suggestions on creating a positive sexual culture around individuals with learning disabilities.

Having said that, it is clear that we are left with a broad range of sexual behaviour which creates problems for services and for the individuals concerned in different ways. 'Difficult' is not an objective word and it is usually applied to situations in which a person's sexual behaviour is unacceptably impinging on others. We would want to be clear that people, whether they are staff, other service users or members of the public are entitled to protection from such behaviour and that people with learning disabilities whose sexual behaviour crosses acceptable limits are not helped by a strategy of ignoring the problem until it goes away – it rarely does. Services sometimes avoid the issue by slipping into a victim-blaming stance which implicates the person who has been on the receiving end of the difficult behaviour, especially if they are young or inexperienced staff or service users, particularly in older, institutional services where sexual exploitation was widespread but unacknowledged. Problems which may have been hidden in institutional settings are becoming more explicit as people move out of large, segregated settings, and are encouraged to be assertive and to enlist advocates to act on their behalf. Community services will sometimes need to acknowledge and respond to a basic conflict of interest between service users who are 'perpetrators' of difficult sexual behaviour and those who are 'victims' of it.

Meanwhile community settings continue to mask such problems by discounting the significance of unwanted sexual behaviour for the victim (Brown and Craft 1989; Turk and Brown 1992). For example a young man suffering from a mood disorder was known to have raped a fellow resident in the hostel in which he lived. Staff focused their attention on this young man, on what should be done to ensure that he did not repeat his behaviour in public, on reassessing his medication and so on; at no time did they consider the victim of his behaviour – the incident was not even recorded on his file. Thus this behaviour was only contained because the victim concerned had severe learning difficulties.

Despite reluctance on the part of services to acknowledge and record such instances, results from a recent survey of reported sexual abuse (Turk and Brown 1992) showed that of 120 people with learning difficulties reported as having been the victim of sexual abuse in the years and 1989–1990, in one Regional Health Authority (serving a general population of 3,658,200) 43 were abused by other service users. Most of this abuse consisted of contact abuse (39 out of 43) and in 21 cases (almost half) the assault involved penetration or attempted penetration. People were mainly abused in residential or day services and like the general public were unlikely to have been abused in public and by strangers, making this clearly an issue where services have to take some responsibility. The victims of abuse of one service user by another were predominantly women in the ratio of 2:1, men victims occurring slightly more than in the whole sample of people abused by handicapped and non-handicapped perpetrators. In 25 cases it was left to the service user who had been abused to raise the issue with only 10 cases being picked up by residential staff. All of the perpetrators were men. This information was gathered in the context of a survey of people with learning disabilities who had been the victim rather than the perpetrator of sexual abuse, and is therefore an inadequate measure of the incidence of difficult sexual behaviour as a whole. Many difficult behaviours are 'victimless' and would not have been recorded and others, for the reasons we have elaborated, would not have been included in the study despite a high profile within local services.

Difficult sexual behaviour is more likely to be taken seriously, when other valued adults, and even more sensitively children, have been confronted by or coerced into it (see also Gudjonsson 1986). A kind of hierarchy emerges, which dictates whether a specific sexual incident will be taken seriously. People who do not have high status such as other service users or young women staff are often not considered important enough to trigger a coherent response; the latter are often allowed to resign as a result of sexual harassment without recompense or support. Such *laissez-faire* attitudes do not only discriminate unfairly but also compound the problems of the person whose behaviour is problematical and reduce the possibility that he will receive appropriate guidance or treatment.

Appropriate concern for the 'victim' of inappropriate sexual behaviour need not, and should not, deflect services from the damage such behaviour can do to the person who is presenting the problem. Whether or not others are involved, difficult sexual behaviour is almost uniquely stigmatising and isolating for the individual concerned. Bizarre sexual behaviours add to the negative imagery which already surrounds the individual and encourages people to distance themselves further. This limits the person's opportunity to be treated with respect or affection. The five accomplishments of services

(O'Brien 1987) make a useful reference point from which to make an assessment of the extent to which difficult sexual behaviour may be hindering or restricting the person's pursuit of an interesting lifestyle and thus underline the urgency and importance of intervening.

Community presence   Has their sexual behaviour resulted in their being segregated in hospital or in prison? Is there a significant risk of this occurring in the future? Are they currently confined to their home for long periods of time – are carers or staff afraid to take them out to ordinary community facilities or locations?

Choice and autonomy   Does the sexual behaviour occupy a disproportionate amount of time and restrict the person's choices of other activities, relationships or accommodation? Is the person excluded from valued activities because of their behaviour? Do they have independent living skills which are not being used (e.g. the capacity to travel about the community freely and independently) because their sexual behaviour presents a risk to others and necessitates a high degree of supervision?

Competence   Is the person's behaviour a barrier to their learning new skills? Does it reflect poor social and personal skills in related areas, such as personal hygiene or communication skills? Does it lead to them missing opportunities to become more skilled at work or through adult education classes?

Status and respect   Does the behaviour lead to the person being seen negatively, or labelled in a stigmatising way, for example as a threat, a pervert or a paedophile? These roles are the focus of very negative attitudes – members of the public tend to hold to a punitive line in the face of deviant sexual behaviour. Within services the person may come to be the focus of lewdness, sexual innuendo and scapegoating which further damages their self-esteem and the respect which is accorded to them in other areas of their lives.

Participation   The role of services is to underpin and create opportunities for people with learning disabilities to belong to a varied social network. Difficult sexual behaviour may present a barrier to contact and serve to isolate them from, or within, the company of others. To what extent is the person excluded from relationships with . their family, friends, staff or neighbours on account of their actual or feared behaviour?

These dimensions help us to put the sexual behaviour in context and assess how serious its implications are, or might be, for the person concerned.

We have, in this section, introduced two distinct dimensions to be taken into account when assessing how seriously to address a given behaviour – that is the extent to which it impinges on others and the extent to which it damages or alienates the person himself. Figure 3.1 will assist services in their initial assessment of difficult sexual behaviour using these two frameworks.

We are, inevitably, mostly concerned with those whose attempts at meeting their needs bring them into conflict with others or are negatively perceived by others on account of their sexual behaviour. Countless others experience 'quiet' problems in that they do not know how to articulate their desires or make relationships which meet their needs. We hope that the frameworks which we introduce to work through seriously damaging sexual behaviour will also help staff to think through ways of supporting these relatively undemanding people. The resignation of people whose lives are devoid of intimacy, pleasure or excitement should be a challenge to services – but it is one which they have singularly failed to address.

Figure 3.1   Identifying difficult sexual behaviour

1. Describe the behaviour(s) you are concerned about.
   When and how often have they occurred?
   What happened and is there a pattern?

2. Are other people being damaged or put at risk?
   Has anyone been offended, harassed verbally or physically, drawn in, coerced or threatened?
   Who is currently being affected in these ways?

3. How is the behaviour affecting the person's quality of life, in each of these areas? Refer to the definitions given earlier and put a cross towards the left-hand end of the line if it is not making much difference; if it is significantly limiting the options open to them put your mark nearer to the right-hand end.

	no problem	------------		gets in way	
Presence	1	2	3	4	5
Choice	1	2	3	4	5
Competence	1	2	3	4	5
Respect	1	2	3	4	5
Participation	1	2	3	4	5

4. Is there a significant risk that the person will be institutionalized (in hospital or in prison) as a result of their difficult sexual behaviour?

ARE WE TALKING ABOUT MEN OR WOMEN?

One of the critiques of the normalisation framework is that it fails to recognise inequality on the basis either of gender (Brown and Smith 1989, 1992), of race (Ferns 1992) or of poverty (Chappell 1992). But clearly in relation to difficult sexual behaviour we have to name the fact that sexual offences committed against others are overwhelmingly perpetrated by men against women (Turk and Brown 1992). It is misleading to report problem sexual behaviour in gender neutral terms (Jupp 1991) since such behaviour is likely to have different origins, different implications and a different meaning for the individuals concerned, depending on whether they are men or women.

Thus it is more likely that men will behave in ways which infringe the rights of others while women who use services are more likely to *put themselves at risk* by difficult or overt sexual behaviour. Women who are sexually active are more likely to be labelled negatively, for example as promiscuous, while the behaviour of sexually active men, even if it is non-consensual, may be glossed over or even viewed as appropriate 'masculine' behaviour.

Nevertheless, we are assuming that it is mostly men who are the subject of this chapter and that their behaviour cannot be understood and properly contained without an acknowledgment of the pervasiveness of abuse by men of women and of more vulnerable men within society at large. This allows us to see such behaviour as part of the 'normality' of men with learning disabilities rather than their 'abnormality' – as failed attempts to meet their needs and control others where other more powerful men might have succeeded.

While this chapter focuses in on sexual behaviour which is perceived as threatening and out of control, future attention must open up the whole issue of how service users develop an appropriate gender identity in services and within the wider community. Meanwhile it is crucial that management make decisions which both acknowledge the relative power of men and women using services, and protect more vulnerable service users (usually women) from those with difficult sexual behaviour (usually men).

WHAT IS SEXUAL?

Because staff work with people in ways which cross typical boundaries, a lot of their involvement with service users brings them into contact with sexual issues. Moreover staff hypothesise about the motives of service users and about their hopes and desires. In short, they interpret a wide range of behaviours as sexual. Many of the behaviours which cause alarm are neither motivated nor maintained by sexual feelings and yet they are pigeon-holed as sexual behaviours and staff lose confidence in the generic skills they have to teach more appropriate responses. There is often confusion about whether the sexual element of an incident lay in the intent, the deed or the consequences, or even whether sexual arousal figured at all. Our view is that services are therefore likely to construe behaviours as sexual on a rather haphazard basis just as they compound the problem by labelling behaviours 'difficult' more or less randomly.

Unravelling these elements enables them to be clearer and more objective about possible ways forward. We have found it helpful to analyse sexual behaviours using the chronological ABC scheme to clarify the relationship between the sexual components and other triggers or consequences.

A   If before the actual behaviour there are signs that the person is sexually aroused or attracted to someone or something the behaviour may be labelled sexual, even if it is later manifested by non-sexual behaviour, for example, aggression or crying.

B   The actual behaviour may involve touching or displaying the genitals of self or others even if the behaviour has been prompted by a need to avoid a too difficult or complex task or some other non-sexual motive. It may therefore not be accompanied by any physiological arousal or sexual feelings.

C   The person may be inadvertently aroused by behaviour which is not explicitly sexual, for example a specific personal care task, or being restrained after a violent episode. Thus the consequences of the behaviour are sexual even though the original intent was not.

Thus, we are not dealing with a clear band of behaviours which we can assume are the direct expression of sexual urges or desires.

This confusion of sexual and non-sexual motivation and reinforcement is echoed in the literature about rape and other serious sexual offences which asserts that sexual motivation *per se* is often secondary:

> Rape, then is a pseudo sexual act, a pattern of sexual behaviour that is concerned much more with status, hostility, control and dominance than with sensual pleasure or sexual satisfaction. It is sexual behaviour in the primary service of non sexual needs.
>
> (Groth 1979a)

People with learning disabilities may sometimes, as individuals, have experienced extremes of humiliation and lack of control/dependency which could lead to a use of sexual behaviour as a way of reasserting themselves. Paniagua and De Fazio (1983) speculate that:

> These patients [people with learning disabilities] often feel intensely envious and resentful of those they perceive as normal. The world strikes them as grossly unfair and they feel entitled to seek vengeful reparation, especially against those on whom they are most dependent.

Hames (1987) reports that in a small group of five young men, who had committed offences, three had 'particularly strong, suppressed negative feelings towards certain members of their families'.

Similarly when we consider less serious sexual acting out, sexual behaviour enables different individuals to effect those around them in very different ways: some may be seeking contact while others are trying to avoid it, some may be seeking pleasure while others are seeking relief from pain. Services need to develop the competence to look carefully at sexual as at other behaviours, to check what exactly it is which is sexual in the events which lead up to the behaviour itself and the events which follow from it. Only then can they begin to make positive plans. Since difficult sexual behaviour, particularly in public, is invariably stigmatising and often punished either verbally, by neglect or even by abuse, a strong framework needs to be adopted by clinicians and service managers to enable staff groups to look more critically at what is actually going on and how it can be either changed or managed.

We have identified four major theoretical approaches which help staff to understand sexual behaviour and contribute to a respectful approach and possible interventions. We see them as complementary rather than mutually exclusive and would argue that an eclectic approach offers the best safeguards to the person concerned and any potential victims of his behaviour (see also Griffiths *et al.* 1989; Crawford 1979).

Psychodynamic	Behavioural
Physiological	Social/sensory deprivation

While psychodynamic and behavioural approaches are often seen as competing theories they both contribute to a model of sexuality as learned behaviour. Seeing sexual expression as learned rather than innate or somehow intrinsic to a person focuses attention on the environment in which and from which the individual will have acquired behaviours that are now acknowledged as bizarre, threatening or disturbed.

DEPRIVATION

Looking at the environments in which people with learning disabilities have lived is an obvious corollary of an emphasis on sexual behaviour as learned. Exploration makes clear the extent of their deprivation from contact and sensory experience. People with learning disabilities may have experience of bonding broken or interrupted. Physical deformities may inhibit touch and holding within the family, and these are notably absent in institutional settings. Mastery and control of food and toileting may not have been achieved so that confidence in being able to take on ways of satisfying oneself is limited and people inhibited from diversifying into new behaviours. Often no models of appropriate intimate relationships are present and people may be confused by those they see on television or specifically excluded from 'normal' behaviour by parents or other adults. There may be covert exploitation or abuse alongside routine neglect or infringement of personal boundaries. Moreover, there has often been no encouragement of appropriate sexual behaviours because of staff or parental attitudes.

A survey as late as 1978 (Mitchell *et al.*) showed that despite the increasing liberal trend amongst academics and psychologists, 31.2 per cent of direct care staff thought that no sexual behaviours, even simple physical contact, were acceptable for people with learning disabilities. The barrenness, lack of comfort, affection or sensual stimulation in institutions, hostels and even some group homes militates against individuals freely exploring and refining behaviours which might lead to pleasure or relaxation.

EARLY LEARNING AND PSYCHODYNAMIC THEORIES

Freud (1905) was the first to make clear the link between early childhood learning and later adult sexuality. He opened up the notion of the 'unconscious' as the repository of all that is learned but not remembered, and defined sexual behaviour as 'a search for some pleasure which has already been experienced, but is now remembered'. His work was verified by animal studies such as Harlow's monkeys who were brought up by a 'cloth mother' and were unable to mate, thereby pointing to the link between early bonding experiences and adult sexual behaviour (Harlow and Harlow 1962). Freud's early theories were made from direct observations and offer a clear analysis of the origins of sexual behaviour which was marred and obscured when he chose later to construct a theory which deflected from the reality of child sexual abuse. Freud describes the 'drive' or 'instinct' for sexual behaviour as having two motivations – pleasure seeking and relief from tension – so that it is both compelling and immensely gratifying.

He outlines the 'stages' of early learning to which these drives become attached, or through which they are developed in physiological terms:

— oral ⎫ these being defined by tissue which is sensitive
— anal ⎬ (erotogenic) and reinforced by the somatic functions
— genital ⎭ of which they are a part

His language tends towards these being seen as a hierarchy, but we can think of them instead as a steadily increasing repertoire of behaviours. Motivation to move from one source of gratification to another is not only internal and dynamic, but external and explicit. Role models, peer group pressure as well as explicit instruction or direction guide us towards exploration of new sexual options. His notion of 'fixation' is useful whether one is using a psychodynamic or a behavioural framework. The person finds gratification through eating or defecating which is highly reinforcing, but if he is then deprived or forbidden opportunities for increasing his options, he clings to what works in an increasingly compulsive way. It is as if he is dependent on one bodily function, on one small ritual to provide him with arousal and resolution.

Freud was convinced that the object to which the person attaches his sexual drive was more or less accidental. The possibility of a sexualised response is common to generalised sensual experiences such as warm baths, stimulating activity involving 'rhythmic mechanical agitation' and muscular activity and the experience of 'mastery' over functions and skills. It is there also in the context of painful experiences, such as punishment or painful medical interventions (suppositories and suchlike) because arousal is the same whether it is pleasure or pain which is being experienced. Because the 'drive', that is the sexual energy, is separate from the 'object' which sets it off, it can attach to things, rituals or certain kinds of people with a kind of randomness which defies blame.

We have been in the habit of regarding the connection between the sexual instinct and the sexual object as more intimate than it in fact is . . . the sexual instinct and the sexual object are merely soldered together.

(Freud 1905)

Anthony has a fixed pattern of sexual arousal from which he does not vary. If he can find a willing partner (or at any rate one who will not run away) he undoes his or her shoes, rolls up their trouser legs and begins to masturbate against the foot. His mother thinks this may have started because a nurse used to bounce him up and down on her foot. However the elements of this ritual came together he now depends on them in the absence of any other social or sexual skills as his sole source of satisfaction, and one which he can count on. Because the sexual climax is so pleasurable, the behaviours are reinforced and become 'fixed' no matter how inappropriate, limited or damaging they are in their effect on the perpetrator or the other person.

As Freud comments, while 'receptive' learning occurs in this way, individuals also learn by identifying with and modelling themselves on the behaviour of others (see also Bandura 1977; Groth 1979b). People learn as 'subject' and 'object', that is, they learn to play one part from experience and the other because they have been on the receiving end of it. This becomes important as sexual 'acting out' is now widely understood as an indicator of abuse and an understanding of psychodynamic theories equips staff to observe the signs of sexualised behaviour which might indicate trauma or abuse. Vizard (1989) observes that:

> Unconscious memories may be displayed as active body memories in the form of sexualized play, or passive body memories in the form of psychosomatic symptoms which may mimic or reenact certain aspects of the abuse, for example dysphagia or difficulty in swallowing as a sequel to forced oral-genital sex.

Thus we can see that people learn their sexual behaviours from three main sources:

— through their own haphazard attempts at gratification
— by modelling others, particularly where they have been abused
— as a result of the response which is made in the immediate environment to behaviours which are seen as sexual.

We agree with Griffiths *et al.* (1985) who argue against seeing difficult sexual behaviour as somehow intrinsic to mental handicap. They assert that any increased prevalence of distorted sexual behaviour can be put down to poor impulse control, the pathological conditions in institutions and the increased victimisation of children, and we now recognise of adults, with disabilities.

HOW BEHAVIOURS ARE SEXUALISED AND MAINTAINED

Although the origins of sexualised behaviours may be traced back to infancy or rooted in past trauma, it is extremely important to see how they are maintained in the immediate situation. If the situation is boring, masturbation, like other self-stimulatory behaviours, is not challenged by other, more interesting things to do. But the response of others complicates the picture by ensuring that the sexual behaviour, not happening in a vacuum, actually affects the environment.

Various authors who use functional analysis to investigate challenging behaviour (e.g. Carr and Durand 1985; LaVigna and Donnellan 1986) propose that behaviours have a communicative function and serve to assist the person:

— to gain attention
— to avoid difficult demands
— to control situations or other people
— to provide sensory stimulation for themselves in the absence of external activities.

It is clear that the same behaviour (such as masturbation) might fulfil any or all of these purposes depending on the response which the behaviour receives from staff in the immediate setting. Observing the person's difficult behaviour in different settings and under different conditions can help to define a specific response. For example, one man touched people between their legs as a way of diverting demands which he could not meet, and once this had been established the way was clear to teaching him alternative ways of terminating interactions.

But, while assessment strategies can be generalised from work with other challenging behaviours, observation alone may not be enough to understand or intervene. Fantasy provides the inner momentum for physiological arousal and can be the missing link in terms of understanding or treatment. Its importance, as both a trigger and integral part of sexual behaviours, means that the 'private event', that is the inner world of the individual, must also be taken into account. Events in the external world are woven into internal fantasising, but the sequence of events mapped out in fantasy is also imposed on outside reality. We have conceptualised this in terms of parallel and competing systems.

Using an ABC approach which takes both internal and external events into account we can see that sexual behaviour can be triggered by a fantasy or by an external situation such as the sight of someone who is for that person an 'object of desire'.

> Observation shows us that stimuli can impinge from three directions; from the external world by means of the excitation of the erotogenic zones; from the organic interior; and from mental life which is itself a storehouse for external impressions and a receiving post for internal excitations.
>
> (Freud 1905)

The actual behaviour (B) may remain private as in masturbation or involve an imposition of the fantasised behaviour on another. Consequences may also remain private or be mediated by the response of others, thus orgasm is experienced as a private outcome, but the person's removal from the immediate setting also constitutes an external consequence of their behaviour. There is considerable evidence that sexual offenders use fantasy as a way of rehearsing scenarios which they later put into effect, holding on to their fantasy in the face of reality, and incorporating others if they are willing or unable to assert themselves. The importance of the 'private event' in triggering and controlling sexual arousal must therefore be appreciated (see Marquis 1970) and many of the specific interventions detailed later in the chapter involve understanding the interconnecting factors in fantasy and reality which are present in distorted sexual behaviour.

The following schema, (Figure 3.2) with examples, enables a staff team to monitor and chart the aetiology of a behaviour and the competing reinforcement of internal and external consequences. This

Figure 3.2   **Assessing the sexual component of difficult behaviour**

	a	b	c
Private	Fantasy	Arousal/ masturbation in private	Orgasm
Public	an 'object' of desire – a person or thing	sexual behavior involving others	response of others, e.g. gets attention, is removed from setting, disliked activity or demands stop

Fill in each of the six boxes above to chart the private and public aspects of the behaviour. Then take a highlighting pen and mark at each stage which is dominant. This will help you to chart the course of the behaviour and appreciate how the personal experience of the individual and the external circumstances are linked.

	a	b	c
Private	What do you think his fantasy is? How will you find out?	How did he behave when aroused? Describe exactly what the behaviour looked like.	Did he reach orgasm? How do you know?
Public	What or who aroused him? Where or when did it happen? What was it about the person or thing which triggered the behaviour, e.g. the way it felt, a particular aspect of appearance, smell?	How did it impinge on others? What made it inappropriate, e.g. did it involve children, violence or a non-consenting adult?	What happened as a result of the behaviour? What did staff do? How did it end?

scheme goes one stage further than that of Langevin (1983) who looks at what the person is reacting to and how, to include what the behaviour achieves for the person and how others respond. It also modifies the charts used by Mitchell (1985) to acknowledge the contemporaneous private experience of the individual.

Observation cannot reliably furnish staff with detailed knowledge of another's fantasy life. Sometimes an individual will openly discuss their fantasies, or they can be elicited in a therapeutic setting with people who have verbal skills. Occasionally, and always under clinical supervision, more objective measures are used to assess an individual's fantasies and orientation, through the use of slides depicting different sexual situations and objects. Interest can be monitored by charting the time taken to view each slide, or sometimes through physiological measures such as use of a penile plethysmograph (Wormith 1986).

RESPONDING TO DIFFICULT SEXUAL BEHAVIOUR

The responses to difficult sexual behaviour advocated in this chapter mirror approaches to other difficult behaviours such as LaVigna and

Donnellan (1986) and Cullen *et al.* (1981) in that they represent a non-aversive and constructional approach. In choosing how to intervene the emphasis is not on 'punishing' the behaviour but on enabling the person to get what they need in an acceptable and appropriately rewarding way. Individual treatment along these lines will be one of three areas to be addressed when responding to difficult behaviour because such an approach does not exclusively focus on the pathology of the behaviour and seek amelioration of this alone. Rather, it deals with the behaviour in the context of the person's current environment, be it physical or social, and the opportunities they have available to learn and develop age-appropriate and functional social skills. In addition, it takes into account the systems, structures and knowledge which need to be in place in services in order to promote healthy and positive attitudes and behaviour towards sexuality in both service users and staff.

Following a commitment to the 'least intrusive' intervention means that these three areas can be represented as a hierarchy to be considered in order:

Stage 1   Enriching the social and physical environment
Stage 2   Increasing sexual and social competence
Stage 3   Individual treatment options.

Crisis management must also be attended to at the level of the whole organisation.

If staff can examine these stages in more depth, they may be able to open up a window through which sensitive opportunities for both individuals and future service development can be seen.

Stage 1   Enriching the environment

As mentioned earlier, seeing sexuality as learned rather than innate focuses attention on the settings within which individuals will have acquired their difficult behaviours. Moreover evidence suggests that difficult behaviour is indicative of current problems in the immediate physical and social environment (Emerson *et al.* 1989). For example, where a person is bereft of activity and social contact it may be that they resort to self-stimulatory behaviours, including masturbation. In order that people can begin to relate in socially appropriate ways, their physical and social environments need to be enriched to provide opportunities to relate to others in ways that are purposeful and meaningful. Maintaining family contact, building social networks and supporting advocacy are all important where individuals are at risk of offending (Aadland and Schag 1984). In order to start to develop such environments we propose models already put forward by Mansell *et al.* (1987) and in the *Bringing People Back Home* training videos whereby participation in all activities that are generated through day-to-day living is taken as the norm, staff consciously plan to initiate and maintain social contacts and families are involved both formally and informally (Brown and Bailey 1986a, 1986b; Brown and Brown 1987, 1989a, 1989b; Brown, Bell and Brown 1988; Brown and Craft 1989; Brown *et al.* 1990a; Brown *et al.* 1990b). Systems and structures such as:

— ways of planning and monitoring staff and client activity
— rotas which ensure that enough staff are available at the appropriate time
— individual planning systems which are responsive to individual needs, desires and wants

need to be in place to facilitate these activities happening.

If these approaches are extended to include the sexual opportunities in the person's life, attention must be paid to issues of touch, social contact, sensuality and physical stimulation, along the lines of a kind of specialised opportunity planning. Staff need to programme social and sensual activities into the everyday routines so that the person's tactile and physical needs are not wholly sexualised. Experiences which are sensual and relaxing in nature, such as warm baths, massage, appropriate touch from staff and friends, nice food and so on, should be balanced with more arousing and stimulating activities such as sports, dancing, keep fit, running and walking, music and so on.

Steps to enrich the environment at this general level are unlikely to give rise to anxiety or ethical problems and can be viewed as the foundation stone for any intervention. Indeed we would advocate that all services should strive towards creating participative environments which acknowledge and respect the sexual and sensual needs of service users. By so doing, we would assert they are being proactive in the prevention of the development of difficult sexual behaviour.

Stage 2   Increasing sexual and social competence

A second area which can immediately be tackled is that of sexual knowledge. In common with other sex offenders, people with learning disabilities who have difficult sexual behaviours are known to have low levels of sexual knowledge (see Hingsburger 1987). They have either not been 'allowed' information, or have been unable to discover ways of gratifying themselves or of seeking sexual contact with others. Mitchell (1987) emphasises the particular needs of persons with handicaps for thorough sex education because they have often been given no training in appropriate socio-sexual behaviours and/or have been punished for expressions of interest in sexuality. When learning experiences are not provided or focus only on punishment, appropriate behaviours are unlikely to develop. Assessment (see Leyin and Dicks 1987) of sexual understanding and language will be important as a route into dealing directly with the problem behaviour but may also help the person to bring his own behaviour under control, particularly if accompanied by relaxation techniques (Shaw and Walker 1979).

Sex education and social skills training should aim to give individuals:

— a way of learning about sexual options and of acquiring relevant age-appropriate social skills
— acceptable ways of communicating their needs to others
— a means of expressing their sexuality in a way that is acceptable both to themselves and to others.

(See also Crawford and Allen 1979; Crawford and Howells 1982.) Mitchell (1987) advocates that interventions will be most successful if they include teaching or increasing appropriate behaviours while simultaneously eliminating problem behaviour. She asserts that the goals of any sex education programme should be to:

— prevent exploitation of individuals with mental handicaps
— prevent rejection of individuals with mental handicap by the community because of inappropriate sexual behaviour
— prevent unwitting experimentation which could lead to devastating social and emotional consequences
— enhance self-esteem by providing appropriate methods of self-expression.

Services need to address these deficits by systematically building competence, equipping service users with adequate knowledge and skills to meet their sexual needs, particularly so where the person concerned has committed an offence because they lack 'confidence, experience and knowledge' (Hames 1987). Thompson and Back (1987) reported that sex education was met by relief from a group of participants who had sexually offended; they 'did not feel quite so lonely to know that other men were facing similar problems'. One major issue which needs to be resolved is for services to decide who is best placed in people's lives to teach these skills and also what are appropriate aspirations for the individual in terms of partnerships and experiences. Moreover, this must be settled within the new evolving structures with its purchaser and provider split so that both funding and delivering agencies will have to play their part in making such a service consistently available.

Staff training and support is important in enabling and legitimating sex education in day and residential services and ensuring good staff role models. Thus sex education can be construed as both a proactive and a retrospective intervention. Knowledge of appropriate behaviour will enable service users to avoid putting themselves 'in the wrong' by being clear about boundaries, consent, private places and sexual function and those who have crossed acceptable limits will be able to use it as a way of addressing and changing their attitudes and behaviours.

Figure 3.3 assesses the context within which a person's difficult sexual behaviour has developed and is being maintained.

Figure 3.3 Looking at the context

1. What is known about this individual's life history, particularly the settings in which they have lived, their sexual experiences and any possible abuse they may have suffered?

2. What do we know about the current environment(s) within which the person is living?

   ● Social

   What is the quality of their interaction with parents, carers and peers, particularly its frequency, appropriateness and how positively it is experienced on both sides?

   ● Physical

   How and where do people spend time? Is there adequate privacy, comfort and warmth? Are there aesthetic surroundings and interesting things to do?

   ● Sensual/sexual

   How and when are people touched? Is this in their control? How is sex talked about? Are people encouraged to feel good about their bodies? Are there tactile and sensual experiences in the course of the day?

3. Do staff have:

   ● regular supervision and forums where sexual issues can be openly addressed
   ● consultation procedures and risk-taking policies
   ● training on sexual issues and sexual abuse
   ● access to clinically skilled professionals?

4. Have individuals had any formal sex education or social skills training? Are there materials and opportunities from which they can learn about relationships informally?

Stage 3   Individual treatment options

Clinical interventions will be determined largely by the function of the particular behaviour. Where that function is of a non-sexual nature staff need to use that knowledge to remove the illusion of sexual intent and to teach alternative means whereby the person can meet their specific need. An example may help to illustrate how misleading it can be to label a behaviour sexual when it is serving another function. John, a young man who recently moved out of a large hospital to live in a staffed house, 'talks about "wanking" all the time'. Apparently he asks if it is OK for him to do it, tells new staff coming on duty that he has finished masturbating, gives warnings that he might feel like it in a little while and so on. The staff are very tolerant and understand that John's behaviour is partly influenced by the very 'coarse' atmosphere on the wards on which he lived. Several staff, when visiting the hospital before John moved out, witnessed people walking around with no clothes on, people masturbating in public and ward staff making crude remarks about them. They assume, quite reasonably, that John is expressing some confusion about sexual boundaries and appropriate behaviour, and launch into long and kindly explanations about what is appropriate, where and when. The result is that after several weeks, John has succeeded in recreating the pattern which existed on the ward, where sexual conversation, albeit in a different tone, is the norm. A second strategy is tried where staff respond to John's opening lines, but then seek to divert the conversation into some other safer subject area. It is only when a functional analysis is carried out and John's behaviour is seen as a strategy on his part for initiating conversations, and one it must be said, which has worked very well for him in two quite different settings, that the energy can be put into teaching him some more appropriate opening conversational gambits, rather than risk confusing him with ever more complex discussions about his sexual rights, preferences and so on. Here is an illustration of a person's verbal behaviour acting as a kind of smoke screen: because staff are both anxious about sex and yet want to show that they can be tolerant and rise to the challenge, they have ended up reinforcing behaviour which must militate against John being seen in a positive light by people he meets in the community.

Where assessment has revealed that the behaviour is accompanied by arousal and sexual gratification and that the individual is using inappropriate means and/or people to meet that sexual need then intervention needs to directly and immediately seek to change that behaviour (Fox *et al.* 1986). We again would like to reiterate that this must be done in the light of the two stages outlined above in that environments, skills and appropriate means of communication need to be addressed first.

Designing an intervention relies on the accuracy of observation and reconstruction of the individual's behaviour. Using the public/private chart outlined earlier we can see that interventions can be geared towards either the trigger, the behaviour itself or the consequences. If the behaviour is tolerable in the current setting and not damaging to anyone else the consequences may be the most amenable to change. Mitchell (1985) quotes one young man who exhibited himself in his day centre – this being reduced within one week by a simple time-out procedure – taking him to the toilet, thereby also showing him an appropriate place. Attention from his colleagues and staff had been maintaining this behaviour so that time away from social contact was effective and in this example new skills were also being taught. We would not advocate time out as a blanket procedure, and indeed it can backfire if what the person actually wants is to be removed from a difficult or demanding setting (Foxx 1976). Certainly, with support, staff are able to change their response and to keep to a consistent line.

Changing the trigger or managing the person's behaviour in settings which act as a stimulus to their problematical behaviour is more complex but if the behaviour is dangerous must be achieved. Planning and anticipating likely difficulties is part of the process of managing community services for people whose behaviour may be unpredictable (Brown *et al.* 1988) and resources must be made available to ensure that the person is accompanied by staff who know what to do in case of embarrassing behaviour in public.

The literature on sexual pathology and on treatment options indicates that it is extremely difficult to change a person's fantasies or orientation (see, for example, Gibbens and Robertson 1983). A number of behavioural interventions are available, although there is little evidence available as to their efficacy in the long term (see also Gudjonsson 1986). Often the teaching of non-sexual skills will improve the situation but, because sexual gratification is so reinforcing, difficult sexual behaviours are very intractable. All these interventions need to be introduced and monitored with skilled clinical supervision and involve working with both external and internal stimuli to shift the link between the problem behaviour and the reinforcement of sexual arousal and climax. (For an account of these techniques in practice, see also Griffiths *et al.* 1985; Hurley and Sovner 1983.)

Orgasmic reconditioning   Essentially this refers to modifying sexual fantasies during masturbation. The client is instructed to shift their masturbation fantasy from an inappropriate one (e.g. children) to an appropriate one (which begs the question as to whether adult women should be seen as an appropriate sex 'object' for someone who is finding it difficult to manage their sexual behaviour or feelings) at the point of ejaculation. Empirical evidence of efficiency is scant, but this method has frequent clinical use.

Covert sensitisation   This procedure relies on the client being able to imagine himself engaging in damaging sexual behaviour. Once vivid imagery is achieved, the patient is instructed to imagine an unpleasant scene or event which will inhibit erotic arousal.

Aversion therapy   This technique has been the subject of much public moral and ethical debate over the years, particularly in the early 1970s when attempts were made to change homosexual orientation. The technique usually involves the application of an aversive stimulus, for example electric shocks or nausea-inducing drugs, in association with the fantasy of the sexually variant behaviour (see Maletzky 1974 for an example in which a foul smelling substance was used alongside the fantasised behaviour). Essentially the paradigm in operation here is one of punishment which would clearly be considered a very last resort in the model presented in this chapter.

The aim of all these interventions is to lessen the possibility of the client acting out his deviant sexual fantasy. Because fantasy can act as a 'rehearsal', changing, interrupting or replacing it with another which will not damage the individual or a potential victim is important. In managing the difficult decisions about intervening at this level, professionals should have recourse to an ethics committee or other consultative group and in making judgements about appropriate strategies they should consider their primary client to be any potential victim(s) (Parsons 1984).

1   Pharmacological interventions

The drugs used in this instance are primarily those which reduce sex drive. A review of the literature by Crawford (1981) suggests that the antiandrogen drug cyproterone acetate and the use of the hormone oestrogen have proved effective in reducing the frequency of sexual thoughts and sexual activity in men who exhibit sexual interest in children. Both these drugs are known to have side effects such as the development of female secondary characteristics. The results of long-term administration are not known and may be irreversible. Before this response is considered there has to be a clear understanding of the function of the behaviour. For example, Crawford (1981) points out that for many paedophiles the attraction to children is not primarily sexual, and therefore another response may be more appropriate.

2 Psychodynamic interventions

Most of the published work carried out within this framework has been related to the area of abuse and the effects of such experiences on behaviour. Valerie Sinason at the Tavistock Institute has pioneered psychotherapeutic work with people who have learning disabilities. Her clinical material draws attention to the use of secondary handicaps as a means of protection if one has been or is still the victim of sexual abuse. In validating hidden abuse, the person is able to rehearse being assertive, and to learn to communicate using skills which do not rely on enactment or identification with the aggressor (Sinason 1989).

Figure 3.4 (see pp. 74–5) leads services through the steps of designing an intervention.

SERVICE COMPETENCIES AND STRUCTURES

Any individual treatment must include strategies for crisis management. Staff need to be confident that when incidents do occur they can respond to them in a way which retains the individual's dignity and protects him or her and others from harm.

Staff who have direct client contact are key people in determining the lifestyle of service users. Their attitudes and behaviour towards clients' sexuality will ultimately determine how clients perceive and value themselves. Yet, despite being charged with this responsibility they often receive the least amount of training, support and direction in how to carry out the work that is required of them. Training in sexuality is now available from a number of agencies (including the Family Planning Association, British Institute of Learning Disabilities and SPOD) but this area is still taboo enough to be overlooked in many services, or to be tackled on the basis of an individual member of staff's interest rather than as a strategic need for service competence in this area.

Both managers and staff need to be clear about their responsibilities in relation to individuals who have a history of difficult sexual behaviour. They need:

— an understanding of the early origins of distorted sexual behaviour so that they can respond without blame

— an understanding of functional analysis which will enable them to desexualise behaviours which are serving a non-sexual function and teach alternative ways of meeting what are essentially ordinary needs

— skills and resources to increase the sexual knowledge of individuals with learning disabilities through sex education and individual counselling

— clear boundaries between staff/care-givers and clients in all areas of practice so that privacy and consent are respected in the course of personal care tasks

— commitment to protect all service users from abuse, exploitation or humiliation, whether they are at risk from members of the public, staff or fellow service users

Figure 3.4   Designing an intervention

By changing the environment and teaching people adequate skills it may be possible for the person to meet their needs in ways which do not bring them into conflict with others.

1. What plans can you make to enrich the environment?

   - social
   - physical
   - sexual/sensual

2. What plans do you have for sex education and social skills training for this individual?

   - Individual and/or group sessions
   - Who will take responsibility for it?
   - What materials/approaches will be used?
   - What support will be needed to do this work and who will provide it?

3. Do a thorough functional analysis to ascertain what the behaviour is saying (see LaVigna and Donnellan 1986). If the behaviour is less 'sexual' than it seemed adopt a consistent strategy to teach the person alternative ways of communicating their needs.

   Check for:

   - boredom
   - wanting to 'escape' from stressful situations/demands
   - wanting contact with others.

4. Where the behaviour is clearly sexual look back at [Fig. 3.3] and consider the potential for change in each of the boxes you have highlighted with your colleagues to see if you can identify the easiest area in which to intervene or interrupt the course of the behaviour.

	a	b	c
Private	Is the fantasy appropriate even though the behaviour may not be? If yes look at b. If the fantasy involves children, fetish objects which cause harm, or violence, refer to a clinician for orgasmic reconditioning, covert sensitisation, etc. If (s)he has verbal skills (s)he may be able to benefit from psychotherapy	If the behaviour only involves the individual does (s)he know how and where to do it? If not can you teach/ show them?	If you have reason to believe that the behaviour is connected to a dangerous fantasy how can you interrupt it before (s)he reaches orgasm? If the behaviour does not seem to be linked to a dangerous fantasy and is not damaging to the person themselves, can it be made more satisfying and pleasurable, decreasing the likelihood that (s)he will inappropriately involve someone else?
Public	What exactly turned him/her on? If it was a person, what was it about them; age, sex, appearance, touch, etc? Can you avoid situations in which this trigger is present? E.g. go another way home, change shift patterns for a particular member of staff, etc.	Did her/his sexual behaviour involve: a) a child b) violence c) a non-consenting adult d) the wrong place? If it was out of ignorance can you teach her/him to discriminate appropriate partners and places? If not, and the behaviour is entrenched, how will you stop her/him?	What should staff do to minimise damage to the public or to this individual? Draw up guidelines for staff about how to handle this person's difficult behaviour in public, including how many people should accompany her/him, in what circumstances they should be vigilant and how they should prepare for activities in public to increase the likelihood that things will run smoothly.

Specify:

- which workers will take on these issues.
- what referrals are appropriate and who will make them
- what resources and support are needed from management.

— commitment to intervene and to initiate treatment through other professionals in order to protect service users from committing any offences as a result of their difficult sexual behaviour.

To do this staff need:

— adequate sexual information themselves
— skills in the analysis of behaviour and design of interventions
— knowledge of the law as it affects sexual offences and people with learning disabilities in particular
— resources to enrich the material and social environment
— proper consultative processes with their managers, and outside advisers to protect their interventions and decision-making
— involvement of advocates and other lay people as a safeguard for individual rights.

Systems in place in services therefore span individual opportunity planning, proper risk-taking procedures and consultation arrangements and a flexibility in staffing resources so that front-line staff can call in extra help in emergencies. Proper supervision and staff

Figure 3.5   Agenda for discussion with senior management/ethical committee

---

Outline your proposed intervention for the client.

What is the rationale for doing this?

Is this the least intrusive, unpleasant and/or stigmatising intervention which be managed?

What efforts are being made to teach the person more appropriate and effective ways of communicating and meeting their social, sensual and sexual needs?

What should managers do to support and monitor the initiatives taken on this person's behalf?

What additional resources will be needed, e.g. staff time, money for taxis, extra sleep-in staff?

Are arrangements for staff supervision, training and monitoring working well?

What arrangements have been made for treatment/support for any victim(s) of the person's behaviour?

What else do you need to know for you to take full responsibility for any risks involved in managing this person's behaviour in the community, eg. present staffing levels and skills, guidelines to staff on how to manage in an emergency? The senior management/ethics committee should be clear that if individual staff adhere to procedures laid down in consultation with management they should not be held responsible in the event of difficulties arising. Senior managers must carry that responsibility.

---

meetings, which address behavioural objectives but also recognise the stress staff experience in containing difficult sexual behaviour, are required on a regular basis so that difficult incidents can be reviewed and learned from.

Figure 3.5 shows how important it is that senior staff practitioners and lay people share in the assessment of risk and in balancing any possible negative effects of treatment with the probable outcomes of non-intervention.

CONCLUSION

If sexuality can be demystified, staff will be able to bring their skills in analysing difficult behaviour and in teaching alternative strategies to their work with people whose difficult sexual behaviour puts them and others at risk. Services should also work towards a positive sexual culture – one which safeguards individuals against the risk of abuse and makes it unlikely that they will be further stigmatised on account of sexual behaviour which, given their own particular histories and the environments in which they found themselves, they had no hope of getting right.

ACKNOWLEDGEMENTS

We should like to thank Glynis Murphy, Tanya Breen, Vicky Turk and Ann Craft who so generously shared their references and ideas.

ADDRESSES

British Institute of Learning Disabilities, Wolverhampton Road, Kidderminster, Worcs DY10 3PP.
Family Planning Association, Education Unit, 27–35 Mortimer Street, London W1N 7RJ.
SPOD (The Association to Aid the Sexual and Personal Relationships of People with a Disability), 286 Camden Road, London N7 0BJ.

REFERENCES

Aadland, R. and Schag, D. (1984) 'The assessment of continued threat to the community in a mentally ill offender program'. *Journal of Criminal Justice* 12: 81–6.
Bandura, A. (1977) *Social Learning Theory*. New Jersey: Prentice Hall.
Breen, T. and Turk, V. (in preparation) 'Sexual offending behaviour by people with learning disabilities: prevalence and treatment'.

Bringing People Back Home, series of video-assisted training packages, Bexhill: South East Thames Regional Health Authority (SETRA).

Brown, H. with Bailey, R. (1986a) *Designing Services to Meet Individual Need.*

Brown, H. with Bailey, R. (1986b) *Working with Families.*

Brown, H. with Brown, V. (1987) *Participation in Everyday Activities.*

Brown, H. with Brown, V. (1989a) *Understanding and Responding to Difficult Behaviour.*

Brown, H. and Brown, V. (1989b) *Building Social Networks.*

Brown, H., Bell, C. and Brown, V. (1988) *Teaching New Skills.*

Brown, H., Ferns, P. and Brown, V. (1990a) *Supervising Staff.*

Brown, H. (ed.) with Szivos, S., Keyhoe-Clarke, A. and Brown, V. (1990b) *Developing Communication Skills.*

Brown, H. and Bailey, R. (1986a) see *Bringing People Back Home.*

Brown, H. and Bailey, R. (1986b) see *Bringing People Back Home.*

Brown, H. and Brown, V. (1987) see *Bringing People Back Home.*

Brown, H. with Brown, V. (1989a) see *Bringing People Back Home.*

Brown, H. and Brown, V. (1989b) see *Bringing People Back Home.*

Brown, H. and Craft, A. (eds) (1989) *Thinking the Unthinkable: Papers on Sexual Abuse and People with Learning Difficulties.* London: Family Planning Association.

Brown, H. and Smith, H. (1989) 'Whose ordinary life is it anyway?', *Disability, Handicap and Society* 4 (2): 105–19.

Brown, H. and Smith, H. (1992) 'Assertion not assimilation: a feminist critique of the normalisation principle', in Brown, H. and Smith, H. (eds) *Normalisation: A Reader for the Nineties.* London: Routledge.

Brown, H., Bell, C. and Brown, V. (1988) see *Bringing People Back Home.*

Brown, H., Ferns, P. and Brown, V. (1990a) see *Bringing People Back Home.*

Brown, H. (ed.) with Szivos, S., Keyhoe-Clarke, A. and Brown, V. (1990b) see *Bringing People Back Home.*

Campbell, V., Smith, R. and Wool, R. (1982) 'Adaptive behavior scale differences in scores of mentally retarded individuals referred for institutionalization and those never referred', *American Journal of Mental Deficiency* 86 (4): 425–8.

Carr, E.G. and Durand, V.M. (1985) 'Reducing behaviour problems through functional communication training', *Journal of Applied Behavior Analysis* 18: 111–26.

Chappell, A. (1992) 'Towards a sociological critique of the normalisation principle'. *Disability, Handicap and Society* 7 (1): 35–53.

Crawford, D. (1979) 'Modification of deviant sexual behaviour: the need for a comprehensive approach', *British Journal of Medical Psychology* 52: 151–6.

Crawford, D. (1981) 'Treatment approaches with paedophiles', in Cook, M. and Howells, K. (eds) *Adult Sexual Interest in Children.* London: Academic Press.

Crawford, D. and Allen, J. (1979) 'A social skills training programme with sex offenders', in Cook, M. and Wilson, G. (eds) *Love and Attraction.* Oxford: Pergamon.

Crawford, D. and Howells, K. (1982) 'The effect of sex education with disturbed adolescents'. *Behavioral Psychotherapy* 10: 339–45.

Cullen, C., Hattersley, J. and Tennant, L. (1981) 'Establishing behaviour: the constructional approach', in Davey, G. (ed.) *Applications of Conditioning Theory*. London: Methuen.

Emerson, E., Barrett, S. and Cummings, R. with Brown, H. (1989) *Using Analogue Assessments*, training manual with accompanying video, available from Centre for the Applied Psychology of Social Care, University of Kent.

Ferns, P. (1992) 'Promoting racial equality through normalisation', in Brown, H. and Smith, H. (eds) *Normalisation: A Reader for the Nineties*. London: Routledge.

Foxx, R. (1976) 'The use of overcorrection to eliminate the public disrobing (stripping) of retarded women', *Behavioral Research and Therapy* 14: 53–61.

Foxx, R., Bittle, R., Bechtel, D. and Livesay, J. (1986) 'Behavioral treatment of the sexually deviant behavior of mentally retarded individuals', *International Review of Research in Mental Retardation* 14: 291–317.

Freud, S. (1905) (1977) *On Sexuality*. Harmondsworth: Pelican.

Gibbens, T. and Robertson, G. (1983) 'A survey of the criminal careers of hospital order patients', *British Journal of Psychiatry* 143: 362–9.

Griffiths, D., Hingsburger, D., and Christian, R. (1985) 'Treating developmentally handicapped sexual offenders: the York Behaviour Management Services Treatment Program', *Psychiatric Aspects of Mental Retardation Reviews* 4 (12): 49–52.

Griffiths, D., Quinsey, V. and Hingsburger, D. (1989) *Changing Inappropriate Sexual Behaviour: A Community Based Approach for Persons with Developmental Disabilities*. Baltimore: Paul H. Brookes.

Groth, N. (1979a) *Men Who Rape*. New York: Plenum.

Groth, N. (1979b) 'Sexual trauma in the life histories of rapists and child molesters', *Victimology* 4 (1): 10–16.

Gudjonsson, G. (1986) 'Sexual variation: assessment and treatment in clinical practice', *Sexual and Marital Therapy* 1 (2): 191–214.

Hames, A. (1987) 'Sexual offences involving children: a suggested treatment for adolescents with mild mental handicaps', *Mental Handicap* 15 (1): 19–21.

Harlow, H. and Harlow, M. (1962) 'The effect of rearing conditions on behaviour', *Bulletin of the Manninger Clinic* 26: 213–24.

Hingsburger, D. (1987) 'Sex counselling with the developmentally handicapped: the assessment and management of seven critical problems', *Psychiatric Aspects of Mental Retardation Reviews* 6 (9): 41–6.

Hurley, A. and Sovner, R. (1983) 'Treatment of sexual deviation in mentally retarded persons', *Psychiatric Aspects of Mental Retardation Newsletter* 2 (4): 13–16.

Jupp, K. (1991) *Seeking the Answers for those People with Learning Disabilities who Sexually Offend*. Kidderminster: British Institute of Mental Handicap.

Langevin, R. (1983) *Sexual Strands: Understanding and Treating Sexual Anomalies in Men*. London: Faber and Faber.

LaVigna, G.W. and Donnellan, A.M. (1986) *Alternatives to Punishment: Solving Behavior Problems with Non-Aversive Strategies*. New York: Irvington.

Leyin, A. and Dicks, M. (1987) 'Assessment and evaluation', in Craft, A.

(ed.) *Mental Handicap and Sexuality: Issues and Perspectives*. Tunbridge Wells: Costello.

Maletzky, B. (1974) '"Assisted" covert sensitization in the treatment of exhibitionism', *Journal of Consulting and Clinical Psychology* 42 (1): 34–40.

Mansell, J., Felce, D., Jenkins, J., deKock, U. and Toogood, A. (1987) *Developing Staffed Housing for People with Mental Handicaps*. Tunbridge Wells: Costello.

Marquis, J. (1970) 'Orgasmic reconditioning: changing sexual object choice through controlling masturbation fantasies', *Journal of Behavior Therapy and Experimental Psychiatry* 1: 263–71.

Mitchell, L. (1985) *Behavioral Intervention in the Sexual Problems of Mentally Handicapped Individuals*. Springfield, Ill.: Charles C. Thomas.

Mitchell, L. (1987) 'Intervention in the inappropriate sexual behaviour of individuals with mental handicaps', in Craft, A. (ed.) *Mental Handicap and Sexuality: Issues and Perspectives*. Tunbridge Wells: Costello.

Mitchell, L., Doctor, R. and Butler, D. (1978) 'Attitudes of caretakers towards the sexual behavior of mentally retarded persons', *American Journal of Mental Deficiency* 83 (3): 289–96.

O'Brien, J. (1987) 'A guide to life style planning: using the activities catalogue to integrate services and natural support systems', in Wilcox, B. and Ballamy, G. (eds) *The Activities Catalogue: An Alternative Curriculum for Youth and Adults with Severe Disabilities*. Baltimore: Paul H. Brookes.

Paniagua. C. and De Fazio, A. (1983) 'Psychodynamics of the mildly retarded and borderline intelligence adult', *Psychiatric Quarterly* 55 (4): 242–52.

Parsons, H. (1984) *The Intellectually Handicapped Sexual Offender*. Connecticut: Ross, Loss and Associates.

Shaw, W. and Walker, C.E. (1979) 'Use of relaxation in the short term treatment of fetishistic behaviour: an exploratory case study', *Journal of Pediatric Psychology* 4 (4): 403–7.

Sinason, V. (1989) 'Uncovering and responding to sexual abuse in psycho-therapeutic settings', in Brown, H. and Craft, A. (eds) *Thinking the Unthinkable: Papers on Sexual Abuse and People with Learning Difficulties*. London: Family Planning Association.

Thompson, M. and Back, T. (1987) 'Counselling sessions for sexual offenders prove useful', *Social Work Today* 18 (41): 9–10.

Turk, V. and Brown, H. (1992) 'The sexual abuse of adults with learning disabilities: results of a two-year incidence survey', *Mental Handicap Research* June.

Vizard, E. (1989) 'Child sexual abuse and mental handicap: a child psychiatrist's perspective', in Brown, H. and Craft, A. (eds) *Thinking the Unthinkable: Papers on Sexual Abuse and People with Learning Difficulties*. London: Family Planning Association.

Wormith, J. (1986) 'Assessing deviant sexual arousal: physiological and cognitive aspects', *Advanced Behavioral Research and Therapy* 101–37.

4 Sex education in the multiracial society

Carol Baxter

The world is racially and culturally diverse. This fact is widely reflected in most towns and cities in the Western world. Staff in health and welfare services are working with increasing numbers of people from racial minority communities. If professional standards are to be maintained then it is of paramount importance that services are offered from a multiracial/multicultural perspective. What this means in practice is that those providing services must have the appropriate attitudes, knowledge and skills to enable them to meet the needs of individual service users regardless of racial origin or cultural background.

In preparation for this chapter I carried out a review of all the sex education material held in an inner-city Health Authority Health Education Department. Although one in six of the population of this area is of either Afro-Caribbean or Asian background there was a distinct absence of material which addressed this in its content. In the relatively few resources where multiracial imagery was used, only Afro-Caribbean images were depicted and there was no portrayal of people of Asian backgrounds. Compton (1989) in her review of models of multicultural sex education highlights their cultural insensitivity particularly to Muslims, and suggests that therapists and health educators may well be perpetrating inappropriate approaches in discussion and treatment of sexuality with students and clients.

Service providers are not always aware of the ideologies which shape their beliefs and subsequently their responses to those they care for and support. It is becoming increasingly recognised that the prerequisite for effective sex education with people with learning disabilities is an awareness and understanding of one's own attitudes, beliefs and practices regarding sexuality and equally important, towards people with learning disabilities. The double discrimination which occurs when a person is also black has received little attention.

The issue of racism which forms part of both unconscious and conscious ideology in Western societies cannot be ignored. A third dimension, that of professional attitudes, beliefs and practices towards people who are black or from racial minority communities, must therefore be explored.

This chapter explores some of the historical and social assumptions which relate to sexuality and black communities. It reviews the value and dangers of cultural information and offers teachers some starting points for improving their professional practice in teaching and counselling people with learning disabilities and their families from racial minority communities.

RACISM AND SEXUAL STEREOTYPING

Black and racial minority people have consistently been under-represented among health and social service users. Whilst there may be instances of personal racism most people working in the caring services would not deliberately withhold services or treat people differently on the basis of their colour. One major explanation of under-utilisation of services is institutional racism which encourages a 'colour blind approach' and ignores the impact of prejudice and discrimination in society.

There is not the space here to embark upon a detailed discussion about what racism is. For a fuller understanding the reader is directed to the further reading suggested at the end of this chapter. A brief overview is presented here.

Racism is an ideology and institution developed out of imperialism. Westerners needed to see African and Asian peoples as inferior and even subhuman in order to justify the gross exploitation and mistreatment which was perpetuated during slavery and colonisation. As a result of this disastrous relationship between black and white people, black people who live in the Western white world continue to be seen through this myth and to be discriminated against. This discrimination is perpetuated by the social, economic and political power wielded by white people.

A survey of people in Britain carried out in 1985 found that just under 90 per cent thought that there is prejudice against black and Asian people. Thirty five per cent admitted that they themselves are prejudiced and 42 per cent thought the situation is getting worse (Jowell *et al.* 1986).

One of the expressions of racism is stereotyping. As with prejudice against people with learning disabilities there is a multiplicity of bizarre and contradictory sexual emotions underpinning the ideology of racism. Sexual stereotyping and prejudice have emerged as a constant variable of racism. Black men and women have become objects onto which all kinds of concocted sexual derangements and myths are projected. The racist stereotype of the strong sexual desire of black people parallels the popularly held belief about people with learning disabilities (Baxter 1990). These views made it easier for black women to be sexually exploited. Historical evidence from slavery in the Caribbean and the United States as well as imperialism during the rule of the British Raj in India demonstrates the treatment of black women as sex objects who were subjected to various forms of sexual violation.

Today a great deal of molestation of disabled children occurs in children's homes and day care centres (Driver and Droisen 1989). Black children are over-represented in this sector. Because of their low self-esteem engendered by racism many may well believe that what is happening to them is part of the scheme of things. The pressures and prejudices of racism, however, make it difficult for black people to ask for assistance or get appropriate help from the law or caring professions. For example, black women are especially unlikely to report rape, from fear of an unsympathetic response and, where the offender is also black, a wish to protect all black men from victimisation by white society.

The pervasiveness of racism makes it very easy for people in the caring professions to reinforce negative stereotypes and perpetuate distorted assumptions.

Unconsciously or otherwise, all the above factors influence some of professional practice today. A black worker at an Adult Training Centre recently told me that the practice of teaching boys to masturbate in private is used in a punitive way with Afro-Caribbean males. They are denied the 'privilege' of masturbating because the therapist felt 'these boys did it too much' and felt that her denial would 'help to regulate them'.

Service providers who have negative feelings about mixed race relationships may put obstacles in the way of the couple and offer little support, as the two stories below demonstrate:

Calville, a thirty-four year-old Afro-Caribbean man with mild learning disabilities has been involved in a relationship with Beatrice, a white woman, for some months. He lives in a hostel and finds that life there is not supportive of his relationship. His self-respect is continually being undermined by staff and the institution's regime. Beatrice is not allowed to come into his room, yet he says he has no money to take her out. Besides these difficulties (which he has in common with many other people) he is also facing personal racism due to his relationship with a white woman. He says people have asked 'Why are you going out with her?' Beatrice's family have also made it clear to them they do not approve. She has been told to stop going out with him.

Pauline, an Afro-Caribbean woman lives in a hostel. It is an all-white environment where she has had little contact with other black people. The staff are all white and have made no attempt to provide a black perspective to hostel life. Pauline has a strong relationship with a white man and they intend to get married. However, their relationship has not been supported by professionals who view their plans to get married negatively.

(Baxter *et al.* 1990)

As products of a racist society all people involved in providing services need to think about the following:

— What are your own attitudes towards people who are black or from racial minority groups?
— What means are available to you to learn about and understand the nature of racism and how it affects your work practice?
— Have you had an opportunity to attend workshops on antiracist practices?
— Is your relationship with black service users influenced by commonly held racist stereotypes?
— Do you address the area of racial and sexual stereotyping in your teaching and counselling with service users?

THE IMPACT OF CULTURE

The concept of sexuality relates to how people express themselves as males and females. This is culturally defined and influenced by family, peers, religion, the law, customs, knowledge and economics. To ensure that education activities reflect the needs of the individual it is important to be aware of the impact of one's own cultural sexual norms and be careful not to impose one's own views, experiences and expectations.

Some areas which constantly cause difficulties for black service users and their families are professional attitudes to premarital sex, contraception, marriage and the role and function of the family.

Premarital sex

The question of sex before marriage has been a moral one for most communities. Attitudes in Britain are gradually changing from moral objections to emphasis on the element of advice, individual responsibility and decision based on a positive self-esteem. The reason that some black (especially Afro-Caribbean) families in Britain may adopt a puritanical approach to child-rearing is to protect their children from the racial stereotype of being sexually loose. For some Asian families, family honour will be a major concern, as the following extract makes clear:

> Girls and young women are regarded as extremely vulnerable in many societies. Members of the family may feel it is their duty to protect unmarried daughters and sisters, and to ensure that their reputation is spotless. Boys and girls may be segregated from puberty to prevent any encouragement to premarital sexual activity. The reputation of a whole family and of all its members may be ruined if one of its daughters is thought to be unruly or promiscuous. Older brothers and male relatives may have a particular responsibility for young women and may act as chaperones if a girl wishes to go out. In Britain many Asian families, for example, feel that their daughter's morals are threatened by what they see as the generally lax moral standards of wider society, and by pressure from their peers to have boyfriends and go out to discos, youth clubs and parties. Some families may become particularly strict because of the increased dangers in Britain, recognising the additional pressures their daughters are under and wishing to protect them. Health workers from a different background may regard this as repressive and as depriving a young woman of her normal and natural freedoms. Such judgements are very much influenced by one's own culture and beliefs and must be made with care. A confrontation with parents over the way they wish to bring up their children is likely to be extremely counterproductive for everyone concerned.
>
> (Mares *et al*. 1985)

Based on the premise that giving children information about sex will encourage them to experiment, factors such as the ones mentioned above may cause some black families to be wary of sex education given outside the family.

Contraception

All the established religions of the world have been, and are still inclined to be pro-natalist, anti-abortion and anti-sterilisation. Attitudes are gradually changing and usually only the more orthodox within any religion will object to the use of contraception. Limiting the number of children in a family to about two is the norm for white British families. The average size of black families in the UK is becoming smaller, reflecting the trend in the white community.

We find a parallel in the treatment of black women and women with learning disabilities arising from anxieties concerning the perceived need for control of fertility. Fears about the degeneration of the race, fuelled by the eugenics movement in the USA and Britain led to the preferential admission to segregated institutions and/or the sterilisation of women with a mental handicap who were of child-bearing age. Bryan *et al.* (1985) in their book on the experiences of black women, comment:

> Our abuse at the hands of the Family Planning service is intensified even further by the many popular racist myths and stereotypes which abound about Black women's sexuality, enshrined within medical science. Black women's ability to reproduce has come to be viewed as a moral flaw, to be frowned upon and controlled – so much so that doctors frequently take it upon themselves to exercise control over our fertility in the interests of (white) society. The consequences of this are evident in the numerous cases of Black women who receive unwanted sterilisations or terminations, or the damaging long-term contraceptive Depo Provera, all in the interests of controlling the numbers of 'unwanted' Black babies. The fact that we may not view our unplanned children in this way within our own culture is of no consequence in a society where we are expected to conform to indigenous attitudes. Many paternal and apparently sympathetic doctors have persuaded Black women to accept an abortion or contraceptive she did not really want, out of a concern to control our fertility. And such attitudes are reflected not only through our experiences here in Britain, but in our countries of origin, where myths about the need for population control are used as an excuse for the unleashing of mass sterilisation and birth control programmes on Black and Third World women, often as part of the West's 'aid' package.
>
> (Bryan *et al.* 1985)

Marriage and parenthood

All parents wish their children to marry someone with whom they will be happy. In some families, however, aspects such as family background and the personalities of the couple are viewed as a stronger basis for marriage than love, romance and individual choice as espoused/idealised by most Westerners. The choice of partner may therefore be made by parents and other more experienced people within the families in consultation with the couple.

> In class in Southall the natives were arguing with the Pakistani and Indian immigrants that the only basis for marriage was romantic love. I took the side of the Pakistanis who produced a shattering piece of evidence – 'But the Queen had an arranged marriage, didn't she!' which reduced the natives to silence. One could argue that the purveyors of romance deprave rather more than the purveyors of pornography; someone somewhere is not taking equal concern for the needs and feelings of others.
>
> (Milne and Hardy 1976)

The great resistance to marriage for people with learning disabilities by both the public and families is gradually being challenged, slowly giving way to more sensitive services. This degree of resistance has not always been evident among some black families. For instance, in many Asian families, whilst the difficulties imposed on a marriage by the mental handicap of one of the partners are recognised, there is not always the same underlying taboo.

Children planned or unplanned are also valued for the enrichment they bring to a family. The added financial responsibilities may have less emphasis placed upon them than in white families. The wider family may wish their member with learning disabilities to succeed in marriage and parenthood, and offer active support and encouragement.

The role and function of the family

Working with families

Families mean different things to different people. To work effectively with families, professionals first have to be aware of and analyse their own preconceptions and deeply held cultural beliefs about what constitutes a family. Skills in working with families are very important but are often lacking in services which are individual centred. Such skills are important when working with people with learning disabilities since many will have to rely on family members and others to speak on their behalf.

The nuclear family has become the norm in Western society and individualism is highly valued. In many families from minority communities wider family networks, including extended family systems, are part of the norm. It may be that the views of important members of the family will have to be sought on issues such as counselling and advice on matters pertaining to sexual relations. Excluding such people could well lead to isolation of the individual client concerned.

Conventions may differ about what is appropriate to be discussed outside the family and there may well also be differences about what is acceptable to be discussed between men and women. Religious requirements for modesty may make it necessary to have counsellors of the same sex and to have single sex sessions. These issues if handled sensitively will engender trust and confidence between families and the services.

One course of action which many service providers have found it easiest to follow has been to focus on issues of language, religion and culture. Even though clients and their families are the most useful and direct source of this information professionals often prefer to look to the vast amount of literature on 'ethnic minority cultures'. This does not enable them to get to know and respect black people as individuals. Whilst some of these materials may be of some potential background value, any information which focuses solely on these aspects will not necessarily result in sensitive services. Much of the information which exists is presented as a series of generalised, fixed stereotypes which does not allow for the fact that culture is not static but changes over time and is affected by fluctuating social and economic circumstances.

A predominantly cultural approach can also tend to emphasise differences at the expense of acknowledging similarities in experiences and perceptions. One example of this is a common response of white service providers to teenage pregnancy in the Afro-Caribbean community. The Afro-Caribbean community is concerned about its high rates of teenage pregnancies and the resulting problems. It is now generally well recognised that teenage pregnancies are associated with lack of self-esteem and poor self-image, impaired family relationships, being in care and the search for economic security. However, the literature when referring to black families ignores the influence of these environmental factors and tends to focus instead on 'cultural differences and expectations'.

There are many shared values and experiences between different communities with regard to sexuality. For example, male domination over women, homophobia and taboos about masturbation are issues with which most communities are currently struggling. Differing views among communities on these issues are usually a reflection of the different stages of development and progress of that struggle.

Bandana Ahmed (1989) in her article on 'Protecting black children from abuse' related the following:

> For example some years back I was approached by a school in relation to a Punjabi girl who was sexually abused by her father and his friends. Although the school was aware of this abuse for some time no action was taken as the 'culturally sensitive school' was anxious to check out whether 'incest' was accepted in Punjabi culture!
>
> (Ahmed 1989)

Such unfortunate responses often occur because professionals are afraid of being labelled racist and opt for the safer position of 'leave well alone'.

The main pitfall of a purely cultural approach is that it locates the 'problem' with the client and avoids looking at one's own attitudes and skills at dealing with diversity.

GUIDELINES FOR EVALUATING INFORMATION ON CULTURAL NORMS

A useful guideline for those responsible for professionals' education is that cultural information *should not be given without first challenging racism and racial stereotypes*. When using material which gives cultural information teachers and counsellors are advised to check on the following:

— Who has been involved in compiling the information? Is it written by someone from the community being addressed?
— Is the material dealing with the culture of:
 an entire society?
 a particular social class or group?
 a particular area of the country?
 a small localised group?
 Is it made clear what section of the population the information applies to?
— Does the material simply *describe* patterns of behaviour?
 • Are these patterns described in a way which makes them seem absurd or bizarre?
 • Does it discuss the underlying reasons for unfamiliar patterns of behaviour?

- Does it suggest possible explanations?
- Is it clear whether the patterns described are ideal or actual norms?

— Does the author make value judgements about the cultural patterns described? For example, does the author's attitude strike you as positive/neutral/negative?

— Is culture seen as a fixed state or a dynamic phenomenon? Is this aspect discussed or ignored?

— Does the information analyse the situation of minority cultural groups in Britain *purely* in terms of culture and cultural differences? Does it make any reference to important economic and social factors (for example unemployment and racial discrimination)?

— What specific new insight have you gained from the information? Has it increased your understanding of the culture described, or created further questions in your mind about aspects you were not previously aware of?

The use of cultural information should be geared towards developing an approach which will enable service providers to appreciate the range of diversity of individual view points and behaviour within communities and to identify the knowledge and skills necessary to plan for the needs of an individual.

From her experience in working in multiracial areas Elphis Christopher (1980) suggests that in one-to-one interaction a person's views on subjects such as birth control, abortion and sterilisation can be openly acknowledged in the following way by a comment such as, 'I know you are a Muslim (Catholic, etc.) and that the decision about birth control, abortion, etc. may be a difficult one. What do you feel about this?' This allows the individual or couple either to reject any advice on the basis that it is against their religion or to admit how far they go along with the teachings of their religion regarding family planning and related matters.

CONCLUSION

Black staff, especially those from backgrounds similar to service users, are vital in providing services to a multiracial clientele. Experience shows that employing staff who can communicate with people in their own languages can result in a dramatic increase in the take up of services by potential clients who are non-English speaking (Dearnley and Milner 1986). However, many black staff feel that their particular perspectives, experiences and skills are often not valued and that initiatives and methods which they develop as more appropriate to the needs of black clients are seen as unprofessional by their colleagues and managers. The majority of black staff tend to occupy low-grade positions and therefore they are very rarely in a position to inform decision-making.

Finally we must, I think, be grateful to minority cultures for sharpening our perception of our own cultural differences without which it is impossible to attempt an equal concern for all who are at the receiving end of sex education and counselling.

ACKNOWLEDGEMENTS

The idea of writing this chapter was developed during a research study on services for people with learning disabilities and their families from black and ethnic minority communities. The study which was published under the title *Double Discrimination?* in 1990 was funded by the King's Fund Centre and the Commission for Racial Equality. Thanks are due to project members – Project Director, Linda Ward (Research Fellow, Norah Fry Research Centre, Department of Mental Health, University of Bristol); Co-director, Zenobia Nadirshaw (Consultant Clinical Psychologist, North-West Hertfordshire Health Authority); Researcher, Kamaljit Poonia for their discussions and ideas.

REFERENCES

Ahmed, B. (1989) 'Protecting black children from abuse'. *Social Work Today* 8 June: 24.

Baxter, C. (1990) 'Parallels between the social role perception of people with learning difficulties and black and ethnic minority people in Britain', in A. Brechin and J. Walsmley (eds) *Making Connections*. London: Hodder and Stoughton in association with Open University Press.

Baxter, C., Poonia, K., Ward, L. and Nadirshaw, Z. (1990) *Double Discrimination? Services for People with Learning Difficulties from Black and Ethnic Minority Families*. London: King's Fund.

Bryan, B., Dadzie, S. and Scaffe, S. (1985) *The Heart of the Race: Black Women's Lives in Britain*. London: Virago.

Christopher, E. (1980) *Sexuality and Birth Control in Social and Community Work*. London: Temple Smith.

Compton, A.Y. (1989) 'Multicultural perspectives in sex education'. *Sexual and Marital Therapy* 4 (1): 75–85.

Dearnley, J. and Milner, I.W. (1986) *Ethnic Minority Development (Kirklees MDC)*. London: Social Services Inspectorate, Department of Health and Social Security.

Driver, E. and Droisen, A. (eds) (1989) *Child Sexual Abuse – Feminist Perspectives*. London: Macmillan.

Jowell, R., Witherspoon, S. and Brook, L. (eds) (1986) *British Social Attitudes – The 1886 Report*, Social and Community Planning Research Team, Aldershot: Gower.

Mares, P., Henley, A. and Baxter, C. (1985) *Health Care in Multiracial Britain*. Cambridge: National Extension College.

Milne, H. and Hardy, S. J. (1976) *Psychosexual Problems*. London: Bradford University Press in association with Crosby Lockwood Staples.

FURTHER READING ON RACISM

Hernton, C. (1970) *Sex and Racism*. Herts: Paladin.

Hiro, D. (1973) *Black British, White British*. Harmondsworth: Penguin.

Katz, J. (1983) *White Awareness*. Oklahoma: University of Oklahoma Press.

TUC (1984) *Workbook on Racism*. London: TUC Education.

5 Sexual abuse of individuals with intellectual disability

Dick Sobsey

Sexual abuse of individuals with disabilities appears to be an extremely prevalent problem in contemporary society. Although it appears that many cases go unreported and remain unknown to anyone other than the offender and victim (Ryerson 1981), reported rates of sexual abuse of children with disabilities and sexual assault of adults with disabilities are high (Sobsey and Varnhagen 1990).

Doucette (1986) found that women with a variety of disabilities were about one and a half times as likely to have been sexually abused as children as non-disabled women. Ammerman *et al.* (1989) found that 36 per cent of multihandicapped children admitted to an American psychiatric institution had known histories of sexual abuse. Jacobson and Richardson (1987) found high rates of sexual assault among women admitted to psychiatric care and discovered that 81 out of 100 women admitted had a history of major physical or sexual assault prior to admission. Sullivan *et al.* (1987) cite several studies suggesting that 54 per cent of deaf boys and 50 per cent of deaf girls are sexually abused as children. Considering the presented norms for sexual abuse in the general population of 10 per cent of boys and 25 per cent for girls, these figures suggest the rate of sexual abuse is doubled for girls and five times as high for boys who are deaf. Brookhouser *et al.* (1986) previously had reported high rates of sexual abuse among hearing-impaired children. Davies (1979) found abnormal EEG readings and active epilepsy in three to four times as many incest victims as in a matched control group. Although there is great variability in the extent of increased risk for sexual abuse of people with disabilities and although there remain some concerns regarding sample sizes and selection methods that make precise interpretation of these findings difficult, the general finding of increased risk is uniform (Sobsey and Varnhagen 1990). Stimpson and Best (1991) interviewed 85 Canadian women with disabilities and more than 70 per cent reported that they had been victims of sexual violence. Of these who had been victimised, more than half had been sexually assaulted on more than one occasion.

Like people with other disabilities, people with intellectual disabilities also have been shown to experience greater risk for sexual abuse. Browning and Boatman (1977) found that 14 per cent (more than three times the number expected) of the incest victims that they studied had intellectual disabilities. Chamberlain and colleagues (1984) report that 25 per cent of 87 adolescent (ages 11–23) women with intellectual disabilities had a known history of sexual assault. Hill (1987) suggests that 88 per cent of people with intellectual disabilities have been sexually exploited. Elvik *et al.* (1990) physically examined 35 girls and women (ages 13–55) with mental retardation and found 37 per cent had clear physical evidence of sexual abuse, an additional 6 per cent had known histories of sexual assault, and another 6 per cent were found to have sexually transmitted diseases. One other resident had an unexplained pregnancy. Thus more than half showed strong evidence of a history of sexual abuse. However, the authors point out that sexual abuse of the remaining half was not ruled out, their status was simply unknown.

This emerging body of research linking disability with sexual abuse and assault leaves little doubt that the problem is a severe one (Sobsey *et al.* 1991). Nevertheless, little information is available to clarify the nature of the link between disability and sexual victimisation.

Traditional explanations of the increased risk for abuse among people with disabilities have frequently focused on a four-stage theory. This theory suggest that: (1) disability results in increased dependency, (2) dependency results in increased stress for care-givers, (3) stress results in frustration and loss of inhibition, and (4) the loss of inhibition results in abuse. This model, however, has not been empirically verified, and the available experimental evidence seems to conflict with the hypothesis (Sobsey 1990a). For example, studies of elder abuse suggest that there is little relationship between the level of dependency and the risk for victimisation (Pillemer 1985; Pillemer and Finkelhor 1989). Other studies suggest that natural families present less risk of abuse for children than institutional alternatives (Rindfleisch and Rabb 1984) and that much of the increased risk associated with disability could be related to exposure to paid care-givers (Sobsey and Varnhagen, 1990).

The mere acknowledgement of increased risk for sexual abuse among individuals with intellectual impairment does little to elucidate the nature of these offences or assist in the development of a useful model for understanding the abuse. This chapter presents data describing the sexual abuse and assault of 152 disabled victims and it discusses patterns within the data, with an emphasis on factors that may contribute to the development of an ecological model of sexual abuse prevention.

METHOD AND SAMPLE

The reports analysed in this chapter were collected over a two-year period by the University of Alberta Sexual Abuse and Disability Project, a study funded by Health and Welfare Canada to explore the relationship between disability and abuse. Requests were sent to a sample of sexual assault treatment centres and disability advocacy groups asking people with disabilities who had been victimised and their advocates to fill out reports describing the offences. It is important to note that this method does not allow for a truly random sample. This limitation was imposed by the covert nature of the phenomenon under investigation and the ethical requirement of maintaining the privacy of informants. Police reports were rejected as a source of data for two reasons. First, many crimes against people with disabilities are never reported (36 per cent of this sample). Second, there is no uniform reporting of victim's disabilities on North American police reports which makes it impossible to identify the population to be sampled.

One hundred and sixty reports were filed, and eight were rejected because of incomplete information, duplication of previous reports or failing to meet the criteria for sexual assault (i.e., third-party reports of apparently consensual sexual activity between adults were excluded). Of the remaining 152 reports, 107 described sexual offences against people with intellectual disabilities (34 of these also had other disabilities), and 45 described offences against people with a variety of other disabilities. All of the reports originated from North America: 88 per cent originated from Canada with the remainder coming from the United States. The offences described in these reports took place between 1971 and 1990 (mean year of occurrence = 1986, standard deviation = 3.7 years). Most of the offences took place between 1986 and 1990, but some older cases were included because disclosure was delayed and the victim was currently receiving treatment.

Data presented in this chapter are from the 107 cases involving victims with intellectual impairment. Data from an additional 45 cases involving victims with other disabilities are presented for comparison on selected variables when relevant to a specific issue. An analysis of the combined data from the larger sample has been reported by

Sobsey and Doe (1991). Probabilities of differences in the distribution of the two subject groups across categorical values were tested by Chi-square contingency table analysis and are presented where relevant.

RESULTS

The offences

Vaginal or anal penetration was described in 59.8 per cent of the reports involving victims with intellectual disabilities. Fondling or masturbation were described in 38.3 per cent. Oral-genital contact was reported in 23.4 per cent (7.5 per cent to the victim's genitalia; 15.9 per cent to the offender's). A number of offences (6.5 per cent) were categorised as forced participation, involving coerced sexual interaction between two or more victims but not necessarily the offender. Some reports disclosed abuse in terms that were not specific enough to categorise (3.7 per cent), and the remaining offences (26.2 per cent) included a diverse variety of other abusive behaviour. Many victims experienced more than one category of sexual abuse (mean = 1.57). The percentages of various offences are similar to those in the remaining 45 cases involving other categories of disability.

Single offences were reported in less than one fifth (19.7 per cent) of the cases involving victims with intellectual disability. An additional 18.3 per cent of reports described two to ten incidents (mean = 2.9). The largest group (52.1 per cent) disclosed abuse on 'many' (greater than 10) occasions, and although they did not specify enough information for further categorisation, the remaining 9.9 per cent described abuse as repeated.

Less than half (40.9 per cent) of the reports of sexual offences against victims with intellectual disability revealed physical harm, which ranged from minor bruising to death. Minor injuries typically not requiring treatment were reported in 21.6 per cent of cases, and more severe injuries requiring treatment were reported in 19.3 per cent. Although a small number of pregnancies (2.3 per cent) and sexually transmitted diseases (2.3 per cent) were also reported, these percentages are likely to be low estimates because report forms did not specifically request this information, and many respondents may not have included these occurrences in their definition of physical harm.

Emotional, behavioural and social consequences appeared to be universal. Although 1.8 per cent of the reports indicated no emotional harm was apparent, these were third-party reports of victims with severe communication deficits, suggesting the possibility that these cases may reflect the inability to perceive these effects rather than their lack of existence. Uncategorised emotional distress was expressed to varying degrees by 58 per cent of the victims with intellectual disability. In addition, withdrawal was seen among 16.9 per cent of victims. Another 16.9 per cent exhibited aggression, non-compliance, inappropriate sexual behaviour and other 'behaviour problems'. These behaviour problems often resulted in secondary harmful consequences such as punishment or intrusive treatment of the victim. Another form of secondary harmful consequence occurred when victims were removed from their homes (9.8 per cent) or programmes (7.1 per cent) as a method of controlling the abuse.

The distribution of these categories of social, emotional and behavioural consequences differed between the group of victims with intellectual disabilities and the group with other disabilities. Figure 5.1 (see p. 98) illustrates the patterns of these categories of effect across the two groups. Withdrawal was less frequently noted among victims with intellectual disabilities, but lost placements were much more common.

In summary, the pattern of offences against 107 victims with intellectual disability described in this chapter is similar in most other respects to the pattern found among the victims with other disabilities in our sample. The nature of the offences and the chronic nature of the abuse portray an overall pattern of severe sexual abuse. Considering this severity of the abuse, it is not surprising that the physical, emotional, social and behavioural consequences are also grave.

The victims

Ages of victims with intellectual impairment ranged from 1 to 51 years old. The largest group (48.1 per cent) was 21 years old or over. An additional 9.4 per cent were between 18 and 20 years old, while 16 per cent were between 13 and 17 years old. Children between 7 and 12 years old comprised 19.8 per cent of the sample, and those between 1 and 7 years old comprised 6.6 per cent.

Victims with intellectual disabilities were 83 per cent female and 17 per cent male. The percentage of male victims decreased with age, with 28.6 per cent of victims 6 years old and under being male, but only 7.8 per cent of victims 21 years old and over being males. This trend toward increasing preponderance of female victims with increasing age was also noted among the victims with other disabilities.

The severity of intellectual disability was not specified for 33.6 per

Figure 5.1 Reported consequences for victims of abuse with intellectual disabilities and other categories of disability reveal more reports of lost placement and fewer reports of withdrawn behaviour for those with intellectual disabilities.

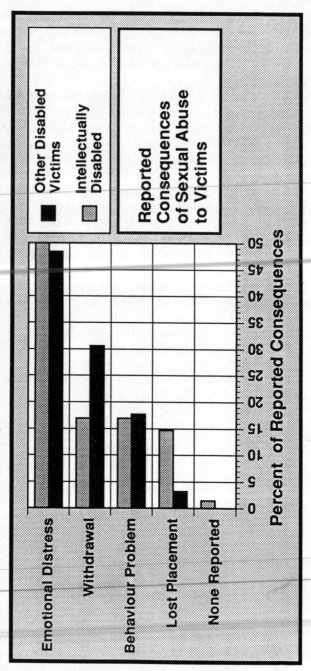

cent of the victims in this category. Of the remaining victims with intellectual disabilities, 29.6 per cent were described as mildly disabled, 26.8 per cent were described as moderately disabled, 31 per cent were described as severely disabled and 7 per cent were described as profoundly disabled. In addition to their intellectual disabilities, many were described as having mobility impairments (17.8 per cent), psychiatric impairments (4.7 per cent), hearing impairments (2.8 per cent), visual impairments (2.8 per cent) neurological impairments (2.8 per cent) or autism (0.9 per cent).

When victims and their advocates were asked how disability may have contributed to vulnerability for sexual abuse, they suggested a number of mechanisms. The most common group of responses suggested that inadequate knowledge or impaired judgement was a factor (31.7 per cent). A lack of assertiveness or too much compliance was cited in 24.4 per cent of the responses. Inability to communicate about their mistreatment was cited in 13 per cent of the cases. Other factors included too much trust of others (8.1 per cent), physical defencelessness (7.3 per cent), the role of diagnosis of a disability in directing the individual to the environment in which abuse took place (6.5 per cent), overdependence on the approval of others (4.9 per cent) and other unique reasons. It is important to note that these responses record perceptions of respondents and are not necessarily valid explanations. Future research is required to test these explanations empirically.

The perpetrators

Perpetrators were predominantly males (88.7 per cent), but some female perpetrators were also reported (11.3 per cent). The average age of offenders was 33.9 years old, with a range of 10 to 87 years old.

In 56.3 per cent of the cases, abusers had a relationship to the client similar to those commonly found among non-disabled victims of abuse. Natural family members comprised 19.6 per cent, acquaintances (e.g. neighbours, friends of family) comprised 13.8 per cent, paid generic service providers (e.g. babysitters) comprised 11.8 per cent, strangers comprised 10.1 per cent, dates comprised 2.5 per cent and step-family members comprised 0.8 per cent.

In another 43.78 per cent of the cases, the abusers had a relationship with the victim that appeared to be specifically related to the victim's disability. Disability service providers (e.g. group home attendants, psychiatrists, home health care providers) comprised 25.2 per cent of the abusers, specialised transportation providers comprised 6.7 per cent, and specialised foster parents comprised 5 per cent. Another 6.7 per cent was comprised of other disabled individuals, typically clustered with the victim in a specialised programme. The extent of risk associated with specialised services suggests an ecological explanation for the increased risk experienced by victims with intellectual disabilities. Ecological models consider the interaction of potential offenders and victims within the context of specific environments and broader cultural influences. This type of model will be explored more thoroughly later in this chapter, but it is introduced here because of its direct relevance to the relationships and environments discussed. If one hypothesises that the risk within natural families and generic community services for individuals with disabilities is no higher than the risk for a non-disabled individual (100 per cent of the norm), the additional risk associated with specialised services based on the percentages of relationships to abusers reported here would significantly elevate the risk for people with disabilities (to 177 per cent of the norm). The extent of this elevation of risk would be adequate to explain most of the findings of increased incidence among individuals with disabilities.

An ecological perspective suggests that the setting for abuse may also be significant. Sexual abuse of individuals with intellectual disability most frequently took place in private homes (58.1 per cent), but it also occurred in public places (8.6 per cent) and other generic community environments (2.9 per cent). Abuse was also likely to occur in group homes (8.6 per cent), institutions (3.8 per cent), hospitals (1.9 per cent), vehicles used for specialised transportation (11.4 per cent) and other environments associated with the victim's disability (4.8 per cent). In total, 30.5 per cent of abuse took place in environments that the victim encountered as a result of being disabled, and this suggests that specialised environments play a significant role in elevating risk.

Only 24.3 per cent of the offenders described in these reports were charged with the offence, and only 8.4 per cent (34.6 per cent of those charged) of them were convicted. Failure to lay charges was rarely the result of inability to identify the offender (3.4 per cent of all cases; 7.1 per cent of cases that did not result in charges). More commonly, it resulted from refusal by the police (21.4 per cent of cases that did not result in charges), prosecutors (8.9 per cent of cases that did not result in charges) or judges (1.8 per cent of cases that did not result in charges) to lay charges. The most frequent reason for failure to lay charges, however, was that the victims and their advocates did not report these crimes to law enforcement agencies (60.7 per cent of cases that did not result in charges). Many of the victims and their advocates indicated that they did not report abuse because they felt it was useless or because they feared retribution from the offender or interruption of services as a consequence of reporting.

Treatment services

The most frequent service sought for the victims of these offences was counselling (47.7 per cent of cases). Various services from current care-givers (13.1 per cent) and medical services (13.1 per cent) were also frequently required or provided. Legal (10.3 per cent) and protective services (10.3 per cent) were sought in a smaller but still considerable number of cases, while abuse prevention education was sought in only a small number of cases (5.6 per cent). Although the victims and/or their care-givers attempted to access more than one category of service in a number of cases, no attempt was made to secure any treatment or support in 11.2 per cent of all cases. Among the victims with disabilities other than intellectual impairment, 13.3 per cent did not seek any services.

Although attempts to secure services for non-intellectually impaired victims with disabilities followed a similar pattern to the attempts made by intellectually impaired victims, there also appears to be some differences. As illustrated in Figure 5.2 (see p. 102), counselling was sought in about the same percentage of cases for both groups, but medical services and assistance from current care-givers was less frequently sought for individuals with intellectual disabilities. Also, legal intervention, abuse prevention education, and protective services were more frequently sought for victims with intellectual disabilities. The probability of these distributions occurring by chance as computed in a Chi-square contingency table is fairly large ($p = 0.073$) when the entire array of services is considered, but it becomes less ($p = 0.041$) when only non-counselling services are considered.

Of those who sought services for victims, many (43.2 per cent) experienced difficulty finding the required services. This difficulty in accessing services was similar to that experienced by non-intellectually impaired disabled victims (48.7 per cent). Unfortunately, even when services were successfully located, they often failed to meet the victim's needs. Most of the services (50.6 per cent) were rated by victims with intellectual disabilities and their care-givers as failing to provide any accommodation to their special needs. Another 10.6 per cent were viewed as inadequately attempting to meet the special needs of these victims. Nevertheless, 21.1 per cent were viewed as adequately

Figure 5.2 Services sought for victims of abuse with intellectual disabilities and other categories of disability reveal greater use of educational, protective and legal services for those with intellectual disabilities.

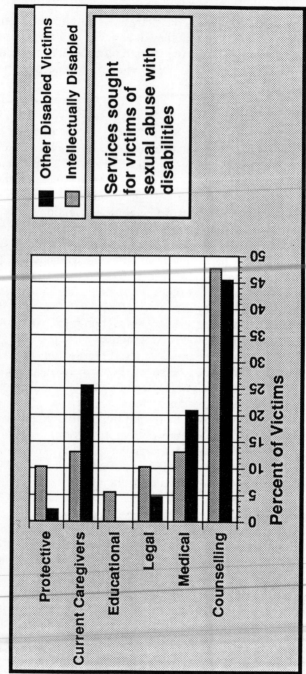

accommodating the special needs of the victims and generic services provided to other victims were considered appropriate in 5.9 per cent of cases. In no case were services rated as going too far, making unnecessary modifications that were not really required. These findings were very similar for victims with other categories of disability.

When the unwillingness to seek services, difficulty in obtaining services and the lack of accessibility and appropriateness of services are considered together, it would appear that only about one tenth of the victims with intellectual impairment can expect to access appropriate services without difficulty, and another tenth of these victims will access them after more difficulty. With further consideration of the increased rate of victimisation of people with disabilities and the social, emotional and physical harm that can result from it, this lack of appropriate services is even more unacceptable. On the positive side, anecdotal information reported through the victims' survey and in other aspects of our work suggests that genuine attempts to serve these victims of abuse appropriately are now being made in many places, and these efforts are beginning to result in real improvement.

DISCUSSION

The ecological model

The results reported previously in this chapter have included little discussion of why people with disabilities are so likely to be sexually abused or what can be done to prevent further abuse. In order to discuss these important areas it is first necessary to examine the previously mentioned ecological model of sexual abuse in greater detail.

Ecological models of child abuse have been suggested by Belsky (1980) and Garbarino and Stocking (1980) and are based on the work of Bronfenbrenner (1977). They emphasise the roles of macrosystems (cultural factors) and exosystems (e.g. communities, institutions) in addition to the microsystems (e.g. families, abuser–victim dyads) usually considered in investigating abuse. They suggest that society's response to disability may be more important than the disability itself in increasing vulnerability and may imply that intervention must be aimed primarily at systems rather than individuals. Figure 5.3 (see p. 104) illustrates the interactive role of offender and victim in an environmental context.

Figure 5.3   An ecological model of sexual abuse

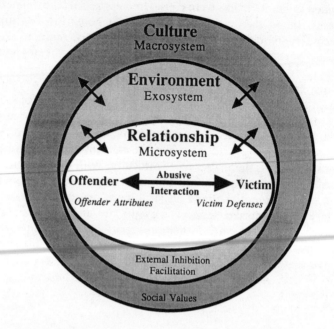

Note: The model views the interaction between the offender and victim in the context of the environments they share and the cultural beliefs that shape that environment. Based in part on the work of Bronfenbrenner (1977), Belsky (1980), and Garbarino and Stocking (1980).

An ecological model considers the role of the offender's and the victim's attributes as influences in the development of an abusive interaction within the microsystem, but it gives equal consideration to the environmental context (exosystem) and broader cultural setting (macrosystem). Of course, the ultimate responsibility for any form of abuse must remain with the offender, but internal and external factors that inhibit or facilitate abuse are associated with the domain of the victim, the relationship between the victim and offender, the setting and the larger culture. Furthermore, the interactional nature of these factors and their domains makes absolute attribution to a particular domain impossible. For example, a tendency towards compliance may increase risk for many individuals with disabilities. However, attributing compliance to these individuals or their disability fails to recognise that families, schools, institutions and other environmental structures have systematically trained this compliance, and it is likely they have done so in response to cultural beliefs that assign low status to people with intellectual disabilities and require compliant behaviour from them. With this model in mind, the following discussion considers some potential factors that contribute to abuse.

The offender's domain

In recent years, considerable attention has been given to abnormalities found in the brains of many sexual offenders. Two types of defects have been given particular attention: (1) defects in the cortex which appear to reduce inhibition (Graber *et al.* 1982) and (2) possible defects in the limbic system (Pontius 1988) which may result in abnormal sexual drives (e.g. an abnormal and intense relationship between aggression and sexuality). A full discussion of these defects goes beyond the scope of this chapter, but certain aspects are important to the discussion. In some discussions of sex crimes, their aggressive nature is emphasised to the extent that they are viewed as crimes of aggression and power rather than crimes of sexuality. While the predatory nature of these offences is unmistakable, it may be equally misleading to deny their sexual nature for the offenders who commit them. For many offenders, the distinction between aggression and sexuality is meaningless. Aggression stimulates sexual arousal and sexual arousal stimulates aggression. Power and sexuality are one. Where such a defect exists, internal inhibition is the first line of defence to prevent sexual abuse from occurring. Thus, some potential offenders may be controlled by their own sense of right and wrong. In reality, however, this self-control depends on the internalisation of external inhibitory factors and continues to interact with them. These external inhibitory or counter-control factors may include such microsystem factors as the perceived defences of the victim and the likelihood of detection and reporting by others, and exosystem factors such as the institutional policies and procedures to deal with abuse or vicarious learning that occurs when observing that others commit abuse without consequences. Macrosystem components, social beliefs, may also influence offender factors. For example, beliefs which emphasise the power of stronger over weaker members of society or support an image of sexual predation weaken both internal and external inhibition.

Offender-related factors which appear to have particular significance for increased risk of people with disabilities include offenders' personal history, vocational selection, social learning and internalised cultural beliefs. Several studies suggest that a significant number of offenders have been abused as children (e.g. Seghorn *et al*. 1987). This history of abuse may act partly through processes described as social learning theory, or it may actually develop abnormal limbic associations between sexuality and aggression as the terrorised victim is sexually stimulated by an aggressor. This association is more likely to occur when victims do not receive treatment. Unfortunately, the high rate of abuse of people with intellectual disability combined with a lack of appropriate treatment services, a lack of appropriate choices for social and sexual expression and other contributing factors result in a significant number of disabled offenders. These disabled offenders are often grouped with vulnerable individuals in group homes and institutional settings, with little attention given to precautions against assault. As a result, the cycle of violence continues. Of course, the best prevention would be to somehow prevent the original abuse of the current offender, but when this has not been done, service providers have a clear responsibility to avoid clustering vulnerable individuals with potential offenders and to protect clients against assaults by their peers.

Vocational selection becomes important when previous offenders choose to work with vulnerable populations. In the course of interviewing victims and their advocates, many reports of previously convicted sex offenders starting new jobs as care-givers for vulnerable people have surfaced. It would appear that these individuals are consciously seeking vulnerable victims. While many offenders have never been convicted and as a result are more difficult to screen out, careful screening would eliminate a significant number; and since an offender is likely to commit as many as 100 offences before apprehension, each offender screened out would prevent a much larger number of victimisations. Screening should take at least three forms. First, police record checks should be used to the maximum extent allowed by law. In Canada, for example, police records cannot be checked for previous complaints that resulted in acquittals, but prospective employees can be required to bring a letter from the police indicating that they have not been convicted and are not currently charged with a related offence. Second, reference checks should be carefully conducted. Many individuals move into new jobs caring for vulnerable people after 'being allowed to resign' or being dismissed for abuse in a previous setting. Often, the dismissing agency fails to keep adequate records of the reason for termination, or the newly hiring agency fails to check with the previous agency. As a result, a pool of abusers can move from agency to agency. Finally, stressing abuse prevention policies and procedures at the earliest opportunity with new applicants may increase their perception of counter-control in the agency and discourage potential abusers from accepting a position.

Social learning also influences offenders. In some of the worst cases, abuse becomes institutionalised. New employees in care-giving settings frequently observe more senior employees or other residents physically abusing, neglecting or sexually abusing vulnerable individuals. The abuse they witness is rewarded rather than punished, and through the process of vicarious reinforcement, the new employee is initiated gradually into abuse. Conversely, in these settings, we see non-abusive employees who resist and report abuse punished for their behaviour. Prevention of this problem is one of the most difficult challenges in the field, but there are many things that will help. First, segregated and isolated services should be avoided. Keeping all individuals closer to the mainstream of community life minimises the risk for abuse. Second, legislation and policy must fully support people who report abuse. Whistleblower legislation or complainant protection acts have been implemented in many localities to protect reporters from administrative, legal and personal retribution. Third, whenever possible, direct service providers must be included in the development of abuse prevention programmes. Stratified administration only serves to reinforce the dichotomy between the administrative fictions and the harsh reality of daily life in an institution.

The victim's domain

Victim-related factors must be discussed with caution in order to prevent the recognition of victim-related factors from being mis-construed as blaming the victim. Among the factors most closely related to the victim are physical defencelessness, lack of know-ledge, impaired communication skills, over-compliance and learned helplessness.

Although not all people with intellectual impairment are physically unable to defend themselves, many (23.4 per cent) of those in our sample had impairments of vision, mobility or neurological function which would impede physical self-defence. The frequent use of tranquillisers and depressive anti-convulsant medication with this population may further impede self-defence capacities. The advisability of teaching self-defence skills to people with intellectual disabilities requires individual determination, but it is worthy of consideration, and generally increasing their physical competence may decrease others' perception of them as vulnerable.

Lack of knowledge or judgement has also been viewed as a factor that increases vulnerability. Teaching people with disabilities to make their own choices in all areas of life, including social and sexual domains, is important. Our data, along with those of many others, suggest that virtually all people with disabilities experience sexuality in some way. Therefore, sex education should be directed towards healthy and personally fulfilling sexual and social expression. It is ironic that when some of the young women in our sample were sexually abused, they were told by the offenders that they had to undergo this as part of their 'sex education' programme. Perhaps if they had completed a more appropriate sex education programme prior to this episode they would not have been exploited in this way. The real question regarding sex education for people with disabilities is not 'if they should be educated' but the question is 'how and by whom?' The decision to omit an appropriate form of sex education from the curriculum of individuals with intellectual disability often becomes a *de facto* decision to allow them to learn from whoever chooses to victimise them.

Impaired communication, especially when combined with physical defencelessness, signals vulnerability to offenders. The perception of vulnerability leads to initial abuse, and the lack of consequences to the offender almost ensures repeated victimisation. Clearly, emphasis on developing communication skills as part of all educational pro-grammes for individuals with limited language is an essential factor in preventing abuse. It is important to point out, however, that communication may be impaired as much by factors external to the individual as those within the person. Individuals locked in isolated residential settings under the control of their abusers with little opportunity to speak to others cannot report abuse regardless of their skills. The summary dismissal of disclosures because we do not believe them or placing a higher value on the statements of 'more intact' care-givers creates the same kind of vulnerability.

Over-compliance in many of these victims not only increases the chance that they will be abused, but also reduces the chance of prosecution of the offender since compliance is often viewed as consent. Many individuals with disabilities are taught that good behaviour is compliant behaviour and that compliance should be generalised to every adult person who chooses to tell them what to do. Discrimination of appropriate times and places for compliance and non-compliance seems to receive less attention. For example, the 'Programmed environments curriculum' (Tawney *et al.* 1979) suggests teaching students with intellectual disabilities to take their pants down within five second of the command 'PANTS OFF', while others (eg Brimer 1990; Foxx 1982) recommend that every attempt should be made to maximise generalisation of such responses by teaching the student to respond to a variety of trainers. Of course, these teaching practices are intended to enable, not to endanger the learner; nevertheless, we must carefully reassess the balance that currently exists between teaching compliance, individual decision-making, and assertiveness. If we continue to educate people with disabilities to do whatever they are told regardless of who tells them, then we are training them to be victims and we are serving as accomplices to the offenders who abuse them.

Learned helplessness may be viewed as a logical extension of this overemphasis on compliance (Kelley 1986). In a number of cases that have come to our attention, so-called behaviour problems resulted in victims of abuse with disabilities were treated by parents, teachers and other well-meaning professionals with intrusive behaviour modification procedures or psychotropic drugs to suppress the 'non-compliant' behaviour (Sobsey 1990b). For example, a preschooler who was sexually assaulted on almost a daily basis by a service provider and began to refuse to go with the perpetrator was treated with an aversive behaviour management programme aimed at coercing her to comply. Well-intentioned parents and teachers planned and carried out the programme. Such programmes can be expected to succeed only to the extent that the programme is more aversive than the abuse. When there is no escape from suffering, victims cease to attempt escape. This phenomenon, known as learned helplessness, has been observed in concentration camp victims and in brutal animal experiments.

Prevention requires that we teach people with disabilities to communicate and exercise control over their environment to the maximum extent possible. As part of these measures it is essential that we make every attempt to understand the causes of behaviour that we consider problematic rather than blindly attempting to suppress it.

The exosystem

The physical and social environments inhabited by vulnerable people also influence their risk for sexual abuse. For example, familial isolation and use of alcohol increase risk. Isolation reduces contact with external inhibitory factors and allows internal inhibition to deteriorate. Alcohol and many other mind altering drugs depress cortical inhibition and allow antisocial behaviour to surface.

People with intellectual disabilities are more likely than non-disabled peers to live in foster care, group homes and institutional settings. Of course, these living arrangements are not inherently more dangerous than natural homes and natural families are not inherently free of risk, but typically risk is much lower in natural families. Not all of the reasons for increased risk in specialised settings are known, but some of them appear to be fairly certain. First, research from elder abuse suggests that financial dependence of the care-giver is an indicator of risk for abuse (Pillemer 1985). This is probably the case because economic motivation rather than emotional attachment (which inhibits abuse) maintains the contact. This does not mean that it is impossible for paid care-givers to truly care for their clients' welfare; many do care, but it is simply not a necessary condition of the relationship. The best solution to this problem may be the support of natural families whenever possible; nevertheless, careful selection of paid care-givers along with the promotion of attachment between care-givers and their clients may also help reduce this risk.

Second, if we assume the same level of risk associated with each care-giver, the larger the number of care-givers interacting with a vulnerable individual, the greater the risk of abuse. Even with today's blended families, most children in natural families are only exposed to a few care-givers, but a child in specialised foster care is often moved through a series of homes and may be exposed to twenty or more care-givers. In group homes, they may be exposed to dozens of care-givers, and in institutions, they may be exposed to hundreds of care-givers. For example, in a typical institution, a residence for sixty-four individuals with forty-eight direct care staff and twelve clinical and supervisory staff and an average staff turnover rate of three years, residents can expect to come in contact with about three hundred and sixty-four staff in their first eighteen years. Thus, a single offender can access more potential victims in group settings, and the risk of exposure to an offender increases with unit size. Reducing the size of residential facilities while working to stabilise client placements and decrease staff turnover will reduce some of this risk.

Third, as previously discussed, some offenders select care-giving professions with vulnerable populations, and offenders with disabilities are likely to be clustered with vulnerable populations in these settings. Thus, the risk is further increased for vulnerable residents in these settings. When abusive counter-cultures develop, the situation is aggravated since more protective care-givers are often systematically weeded out. Screening procedures that were previously discussed are essential for reducing this risk. Cultivation and support of protective staff attitudes may be equally important. A staff truly committed to recognising, reporting and eliminating abuse will radically reduce risk for clients.

Finally, society may be more willing to tolerate abuse in institutional settings than in natural families. In a report of the dropping of 250 charges of sexual abuse against 14 staff members in a Quebec group home (Van Dusen 1987) a government official is quoted suggesting that society would be outraged if the same scenario occurred in a day care or public school, but society's response to abuse in a group home is largely lack of interest. Chase (1975) refers to this 'institutional double standard', pointing out that 'there are far more American children mistreated in institutions than suffer neglect or injury at home'. Changing cultural attitudes and beliefs will be discussed later under macrosystem factors, but again, supporting natural family units and integrating alternative living arrangements into the fabric of community life will help ensure more equal expectations.

Considering these environmental factors, it is not surprising that Rindfleisch and Rabb (1984) found that risk of abuse is about two and a half times as high (and probably higher when underreporting is considered) in institutions as in community settings. This rate, considered along with Gil's 1982 finding that 23 per cent of cases of institutional abuse involve sexual abuse, compared to about 10 per cent of reports in the general population (e.g. Gargiulo 1990), suggests that risk for sexual abuse is as much as six times as high in institutional settings as in the general population. Considering this, environment must be viewed as a powerful force in the abuse of these individuals.

The macrosystem

How cultural beliefs and values may inhibit or facilitate the sexual abuse of individuals may be hard to understand at first and it remains a difficult area to investigate systematically. Nevertheless, our views of people with intellectual disabilities appear to be a powerful force (Waxman 1991). For example, the quality of life of people with intellectual disabilities has been a subject of considerable discussion. Arguments have been raised that the quality of life for people with intellectual disabilities is so poor that life is not worth living, and in some cases these beliefs have even been used to justify ending lives of children with disabilities (Schaffer and Sobsey 1990). Such arguments seem to suggest that the amount of pleasure experienced in life is directly related to the intelligence of the individual, but such a proposition defies empirical verification. Everyday life experience tells us that some intelligent people lead wasted and painful lives, while others who are less gifted lead enjoyable and productive lives. However, for the sexual offender, this myth may feed a second, related myth. Since the disabled victim's life is already worthless, it cannot be damaged further by abuse.

Dehumanisation of people with disabilities conceptualises them as less than human. Viewed in this way, they are no longer entitled to the protection or dignity of other human beings. Wolfensberger (1975) devotes considerable discussion to the effect of this view of 'the retarded person as subhuman' on the development of institutional care. A related myth, also discussed by Wolfensberger, is the lack of sensitivity to physical or emotional pain. One version of this myth permits institutional physicians to sew up lacerations without the use of anaesthetics. It may also be used by offenders. A second version of this myth is used by sexual offenders who suggest that victims with intellectual impairments do not understand what happens to them and therefore are not harmed by it (see chapter eight by Sinason). Such myths are probably reinforced by the learned helplessness displayed by many disabled individuals who no longer resist or demonstrate their pain because earlier cries for mercy have been ignored.

Another myth discussed by Wolfensberger is the view of the individual with an intellectual handicap as a threat to society. This myth may influence abuse in at least two ways. First, since the victim is viewed as deviant, the victim rather than the offender is frequently seen as responsible for the abuse. The distinction between increased vulnerability and responsibility for the act is easily blurred in the minds of some individuals, and the characteristic of victims' behaviour as 'provoking abuse' (e.g. Rusch, Hall and Griffin 1986) may add to this confusion. Second, the belief that people with disabilities pose a threat becomes a major rationale for segregating them from the mainstream of society. Segregation, in turn, further increases the risk for abuse.

While other images of people with intellectual handicaps may seem more benevolent, they may also have dangerous effects. Ironically, even the identification of the vulnerability of this group may encourage offenders to believe that they can act without fear of apprehension or punishment. Also, while research suggests increased risk in segregated environments, abuse within institutions is less well known to the outside world, and well-meaning advocates may institutionalise some individuals to shelter them from better-known risks in the community.

Changing attitudes and beliefs is a major challenge, but three important elements for creating this change are education, experience and advocacy. Public education must continue to provide realistic images of people with intellectual disabilities as individuals and not as stereotyped constructs. Increased integration will provide more members of society with direct experience that will reinforce more realistic views. Finally, direct advocacy is necessary to dispel the myths that support abuse. Each time an attempt to starve a disabled child to death, to deny anaesthesia to a person in pain or to 'protect' a child in an institution is successfully challenged, it helps to defeat the attitudes that facilitate abuse of all disabled children.

CONCLUSION

This chapter presented data on victims of sexual abuse with intellectual disabilities. An ecological model of abuse was explored, with emphasis on examples of the micro-, exo- and macrosystem variables that appear to increase risk and some preliminary steps toward prevention. Currently, there is growing concern about this problem and consequently there is reason to hope that improvement is beginning to occur. Nevertheless, substantial amelioration of such a large and long-standing problem will not occur without a major and continuing effort. While the focus of this chapter has been on the special problems faced by individuals with intellectual disabilities, sexual abuse and assault are concerns for all members of society. No solution can be expected to entirely solve this problem for a single segment until a solution is found that protects every member of society. Perhaps a better understanding of the special factors contributing to the vulnerability of these victims will contribute to the overall solution.

AUTHOR'S NOTE

Portions of the project that provided the basis for this chapter were funded by the National Health Research and Development Program, Health and Welfare Canada, under projects 6609–1465 CSA and 6609–1597 FV. Findings and opinions expressed are those of the author and not necessarily those of the funding agency.

REFERENCES

Ammerman, R.T., Van Haslett, V.B., Mersen, M., McGonigle, J.J. and Lubetsky, M.J. (1989) 'Abuse and neglect in psychiatrically hospitalized multihandicapped children'. *Child Abuse and Neglect* 13 335–43.

Belsky, J. (1980) 'Child maltreatment: an ecological integration'. *American Psychologist*, 35 (4), 320–35.

Brimer, R.W. (1990) *Students with Severe Disabilities: Current Perspectives and Practices*. Mountainview, Calif: Mayfield Publishing Co.

Bronfenbrenner, U. (1977) 'Toward an experimental ecology of human development'. *American Psychologist*, 32, 513–31.

Brookhouser, P.E., Sullivan, P., Scanlan, J.M. and Garbarino, J. (1986) 'Identifying the sexually abused deaf child: the otolaryngologists's role'. *Laryngoscope*, 96, 152–8.

Browning, D.H. and Boatman, B. (1977) 'Incest: children at risk'. *American Journal of Psychiatry*, 13, 69–72.

Chamberlain, A., Rauh, J., Passer, A., McGrath, M. and Burket, R. (1984) 'Issues in fertility control for mentally retarded female adolescents: I. Sexual activity, sexual abuse and contraception'. *Pediatrics*, 73, 445–50.

Chase, N.F. (1975) *A Child is being Beaten: Violence against Children. An American Tragedy*. New York: McGraw-Hill.

Davies, R.K. (1979) 'Incest and vulnerable children'. *Science News*, 116, 244–5.

Doucette, J. (1986) *Violent Acts against Disabled Women*. Toronto: DAWN (DisAbled Women's Network) Canada.

Elvik, S.L., Berkowitz, C.D., Nicholas, E., Lipman, J.L. and Inkelis, S.H. (1990) 'Sexual abuse in the developmentally disabled: dilemmas in diagnosis'. *Child Abuse and Neglect* 14, 497–502.

Foxx, R.M. (1982) *Increasing the Behaviors of Severely Retarded and Autistic Persons*. Champaign, Ill: Research Press.

Garbarino, J. and Stocking, S.H. (1980) 'The social context of child maltreatment', in J. Garbarino and S.H. Stocking (eds) *Protecting Children from Abuse and Neglect: Developing and Maintaining Support Systems for Families*: 1–14. San Francisco: Jossey-Bass.

Gargiulo, R. (1990) 'Child abuse and neglect: an overview', in R. Goldman and R.M. Gargiulo (eds). *Children at Risk: An Interdisciplinary Approach to Child Abuse and Neglect*. Austin, Texas: Pro-Ed.

Gil, E. (1982) 'Institutional abuse of children in out-of-home care', in R. Hansen (ed.). *Institutional Abuse of Children and Youth*: 7–13. New York: Haworth Press.

Graber, B., Hartmann, K., Coffmann, J.A., Huey, C.H. and Golden, B. (1982) 'Brain damage among mentally disordered sex offenders'. *Journal of Forensic Sciences*, 27, 125–44.

Hill, G. (1987) 'Sexual abuse and the mentally handicapped'. *Child Sexual Abuse Newsletter*, 6, 4.

Jacobson, A. and Richardson, B. (1987) 'Assault experiences of 100 psychiatric inpatients: evidence for the need for routine inquiry'. *American Journal of Psychiatry*, 144, 908–13.

Kelley, S.J. (1986) 'Learned helplessness in the sexually abused child'. *Issues in Comprehensive Pediatric Nursing*, 9, 193–207.

Pillemer, K. (1985) 'The dangers of dependency: new findings on the domestic violence against the elderly'. *Social Problems*, 33, 146–58.

Pillemer, K. and Finkelhor, D. (1989) 'Causes of elder abuse: caregiver stress versus problem relatives'. *American Journal of Orthopsychiatry*, 59, 179–87.

Pontius, A. (1988) 'Limbic system-frontal lobes' role in subtypes of "atypical rape"'. *Psychological Reports*, 63, 879–88.

Rindfleisch, N. and Rabb, J. (1984) 'How much of a problem is resident mistreatment in child welfare institutions?' *Child Abuse and Neglect*, 8, 33–40.

Rusch, R.G., Hall, J.C. and Griffin, H.C. (1986) 'Abuse-provoking characteristics of institutionalized mentally retarded individuals'. *American Journal of Mental Deficiency*, 90, 618–24.

Ryerson, E. (1981) 'Sexual abuse of disabled persons and prevention alternatives', in D.G. Bullard and S.E. Knight (eds) *Sexuality and Physical Disability: Personal perspectives*: 235–42, St Louis: C V Mosby.

Schaffer, J. and Sobsey, D. (1990) 'A dialogue on medical responsibility', in L.H. Meyer, L. Brown and C. Peck (eds) *Critical Issues in the Lives of People with Severe Disabilities*. Baltimore: Paul H. Brookes.

Seghorn, T.K., Prentky, R.A. and Boucher, R.J. (1987) 'Childhood sexual abuse in the lives of sexually aggressive offenders'. *Journal of the American Academy of Child and Adolescent Psychiatry*, 26, 262–7.

Sobsey, D. (1990a) 'Too much stress on stress? Abuse and the family stress factor'. *Quarterly Newsletter of the American Association on Mental Retardation*, 3 (1): 2, 8.

Sobsey, D. (1990b) 'Modifying the behavior of behavior modifiers: arguments for countercontrol against aversive procedures', in A. Repp and N. Singh (eds) *Perspectives on the Use of Non-aversive Behavior and Aversive Interventions for Persons with Developmental Disabilities*: 421–33, Sycamore, Ill: Sycamore Publishing.

Sobsey, D. and Doe, T. (1991) 'Patterns of sexual abuse and assault'. *Journal of Sexuality and Disability* 9 (3): 243–59.

Sobsey, D., Gray, S., Wells, D., Pyper, D. and Reimer-Heck, B. (1991) *Disability, Sexuality and Abuse: An Annotated Bibliography*. Baltimore: Paul H. Brookes.

Sobsey, D. and Varnhagen, C. (1990) 'Sexual abuse, assault and exploitation of individuals with disabilities', in C. Bagley and R.J. Thomlinson (eds) *Child Sexual Abuse: Critical Perspectives on Prevention, Assessment and Treatment*. Toronto: Wall and Emerson.

Stimpson, L. and Best, M.C. (1991) *Courage above All: Sexual Assault against Women with Disabilities*. Toronto: DAWN (DisAbled Women's Network) Canada.

Sullivan, P.M., Vernon, M. and Scanlan, J.M. (1987) 'Sexual abuse of deaf youth'. *American Annals of the Deaf*, 132, 256–62.

Tawney, J.W., Knapp, D.S., O'Reilly, C.D. and Pratt, S.S. (1979) *Programmed Environments Curriculum*. Columbus, Ohio: Charles E. Merrill.

Van Dusen, L. (1987) 'We just want the truth'. *Maclean's*: 100 (44): 56, 58.

Waxman, B. (1991) 'Hatred: the unacknowledged dimension in violence against disabled people'. *Journal of Sexuality and Disability* 9 (3): 185–99.

Wolfensberger, W. (1975) *The Origin and Nature of our Institutional Models*. Syracuse, NY: Human Policy Press.

6 Competency and consent
The importance of decision-making

Michael Gunn

THE SIGNIFICANCE OF COMPETENCY AND CONSENT: THE IMPORTANCE OF DECISION-MAKING

People regularly are required to make decisions. The ability to make such decisions is an important mark of a person's independence. It is, therefore, crucial that a person is allowed to make decisions whenever possible and that those decisions are respected. Respect for decisions may involve accepting a decision which is not perceived by others to be sensible. So, for example, a Jehovah's Witness is entitled to decide not to accept a blood transfusion even if everyone else involved is of the view that recovery from a severe stab wound is not possible without such a transfusion (*R* v *Blaue* (1975)). Writers of wills (testators) are not required to leave their property to spouses and children. Although Parliament has indicated that dependant relatives may have a claim on the estate if not provided for (Inheritance (Provision for Family and Dependants) Act 1975), the will that the testator writes is not invalidated by failure to provide for such people.

An adult with learning disabilities is in no different position. As an adult, her or his decisions must be respected, even if they are perceived by others, such as carers, not to be entirely appropriate or sensible or decisions 'which I think are right'. These assertions are based upon the principles of autonomy and self-determination. They appear to be generally accepted principles upon which it is appropriate to base the practice of accepting an adult's decisions. Indeed Cardozo, an American judge, expressly recognised the principle in the context of consent to treatment, when he said:

'Every human being of adult years and sound mind has a right to determine what shall be done with his own body'
(*Schloendorff* v *Society of New York Hospitals* (1914)).

Of course, the position is not quite so straightforward as is so far suggested. The right to recognition of one's decisions rests on a prior premise. A person must be able, competent or capable of making such decisions. With adults this is presumed to be the case. In the case of a testator, the burden of proof is upon the person alleging incapacity to prove it (*Wellesley* v *Vere* (1841)). There is no reason to suppose that a different approach would be taken in any other area of decision-making. If the purported decision-maker is an adult with learning disabilities, it is important to recognise that issues of competency do arise. Whether they should arise, and cause as much concern as they sometimes do, is a matter which should be debated amongst the carers and service-deliverers. There is no basis for presuming incompetency simply because a person carries a particular label, such as 'learning disabilities' or 'mental handicap'. On the other hand, it must be recognised that some people with learning disabilities will be incapable of taking some (or many or all) decisions at some (or many or all) times.

It makes little sense to espouse only the importance of the right to autonomy and self-determination if an adult is not capable of making decisions. This is recognised in the first article of the United Nations' *Declaration of the Rights of Mentally Retarded Persons* (1971):

The mentally retarded person has, to the maximum degree of feasibility, the same rights as other human beings.

Fennell has also made the same point by stating that

[h]ealth care decision-making with regard to mentally disordered people is permeated by the need to strike the appropriate balance between two dimensions of the obligation to show respect for the wishes of the person. . . . There is now widespread acknowledgement of the folly of rigid insistence upon the ascendancy of patient autonomy over paternalism where the result would be harm to the patient.

(Fennell 1990: 29)

Having recognised the impracticality of only relying upon the individual, the UN Declaration goes on, *inter alia*, to attempt to ensure that a 'mentally retarded person' is provided with that support which she or he requires to achieve her or his full potential. This is a vital element of any approach to decision-making. Resolving the problem about incapacity and consent or decision-making is not merely about responding to a specific problem created by an individual's lack of capacity to consent, but it is also about enhancing and developing that individual's ability to make decisions and be independent.

There is a balance of interests to be achieved if there is to be an appropriate response to the needs of people with learning disabilities (and others) who are not capable of making their own decisions. The Law Commission in its recent report (1991) indicated that the following are the various values and principles of which adequate account must be taken in examining the law in this area:

a) Normalisation

The Commission explained this principle as having as its aims

> to treat mentally disordered people as much like other people as possible and integrate them into the mainstream of everyday life. It also encompasses the maximisation of potential by encouraging people who are to some extent mentally disordered or incapacitated to make decisions for themselves, so that they can learn from them and thus attain a greater degree of independence.
>
> (Law Commission 1991: 102)

b) The presumption of competence

It has already been indicated that it is presumed in law that an individual is competent to consent and make decisions and thus the burden is on the person alleging otherwise to prove it.

c) The least restrictive alternative

The Commission explained that this principle has two distinct aspects.

> The first is that treatment or care should be provided in the least restrictive circumstances possible. . . . The second is that preference must be given to the means of accomplishing an end that least restricts individual rights, so that intervention must be the minimum required to provide adequate protection.
>
> (Law Commission 1991: 104)

d) Providing safeguards without stigma

The Commission pointed out that the risk of stigma, which 'arises when others perceive someone to belong to a particular category . . . about which they have negative preconceptions', can be reduced by 'well designed procedures framed in a way which, so far as possible, recognise the widespread reluctance of families and professions to invoke formal provisions'

(Law Commission 1991: 105)

e) The 'substituted judgement' versus the 'best interests' test

The former, as the Commission pointed out, is 'generally thought preferable to the best interests test in principle. [But] applying it in practice raises problems. It is more difficult to apply in the case of someone who has never had capacity . . .'

(Law Commission 1991: 107)

The Commission recognised that some of these principles and values compete with one another and thus a compromise may be required in order to achieve a balance. In consequence, the Commission concluded that

[t]he aims of policy in this area may perhaps be summarised thus:
  (i)   that people are enabled and encouraged to take for themselves those decisions which they are able to take;
  (ii) that where it is necessary in their own interests or for the protection of others that someone else should take decisions on their behalf, the intervention should be as limited as possible and concerned to achieve what the person himself would have wanted; and
  (iii) that proper safeguards be provided against exploitation, neglect, and physical, sexual or psychological abuse.

(Law Commission 1991: 110)

The approach taken by the Commission as indicated above appears to be in accord with the UN Declaration and may be regarded as a reasonable basis upon which to examine the existing law. It should be made clear that the Commission was desirous of establishing what principles and values are of importance in order to assess what, if any, reform is needed. Nevertheless, those principles and values may operate fairly as a measure by which existing legal provisions may be criticised.

CONSENT TO TREATMENT AS AN EXAMPLE OF DECISION-MAKING

The intention in this part of the chapter is to examine the recently contentious issue of consent to treatment as an example of how the law may approach issues related to competency in decision-making. Thereafter other examples where incapacity, consent and decision-making create problems are examined to consider what answers, if any, are currently provided.

First it must be decided what the law understands by the activity in question, in this case 'treatment'. The law has certain headings under which cases can be brought. In order to analyse the legal significance of a particular activity, it has to be determined whether there is a legal heading which may deal with that activity. Treatment involves, quite often, bodily contact by the treatment provider with the 'patient' or 'client'. If the matter of simple bodily contact is considered, the activity can be placed under the legal headings: the tort (civil wrong) or crime of assault and battery. Assault and battery are different legal headings, although they are usually considered together. 'Assault', in its technical sense, has been described as 'an act which causes another person to apprehend the infliction of immediate, unlawful, force on [her or] his person' (*Collins* v *Wilcock* (1984)). 'Battery' has been described as 'the actual infliction of unlawful force on another person' (*Collins* v *Wilcock* (1984)). For many, though not all purposes, these will be the significant headings, in which case it will be important to consider what is 'unlawful force' and when and if there is a defence to such activity so that a person providing treatment is not legally liable.

The essential element in assault and battery is that there must be the apprehension or actual infliction of 'unlawful force'. At one time the phrase used was 'unlawful personal violence'. The consequent impression was that there would have to be some quite outrageous interference with bodily integrity. In fact, no such thing is required. 'Force' means no more than bodily contact. 'Unlawful' means that there is no law permitting the contact. Thus treatment is 'unlawful force' provided it involves actual or apprehended bodily contact. Consequently, 'treatment' can, for legal purposes, be extended to any form of care which includes bodily contact. 'Treatment' has, at this stage at least, no particular legal significance as a concept. What matters, therefore, is whether the bodily contact is 'unlawful'. It is widely accepted that, for example, such contact is not unlawful where it is a part of the 'ordinary conduct of daily life' (*Collins* v *Wilcock* (1984): 378). Thus the jostling to be expected in a busy high street cannot, by itself, provide the basis of a legal action. Such an approach has no relevance to the legality or otherwise of treatment (*T* v *T* (1988), *Re F* (1989)). It has been argued that there is no assault and battery if the contact is not 'hostile' (*Wilson* v *Pringle* (1986)). This would allow most forms of treatment. It is now clear, however, that it is not a relevant issue (*Re F* (1989)). If the legality of treatment is to be considered, there are two defences which may mean that the contact is lawful: consent and necessity.

The defence of consent has been said by the court in *Chatterton* v *Gerson* (1981) to be present when a person understands in broad terms the treatment that is proposed and has consented to it. The competency issue is, therefore, concerned with whether a person understands in broad terms the nature of the treatment proposed. Before considering this vital question, it is important to indicate that consent is not valid if it is not voluntarily provided (*Freeman* v *Home Office* (1984)). Voluntariness may not be present if, for example, the treatment provider exercises undue influence over the treatment recipient. A classic example of undue influence is to be found in the law of wills, where a housekeeper was held to have exercised undue influence over her elderly employer who, in his last will, left all his estate to that housekeeper (*Re Craig* (1971)). Further, consent is not valid if fraud is practised on the patient such that he or she makes a fundamental mistake about the nature of the treatment (see Gunn 1987: 246).

The primary issue for present purposes is that of competency. In *Chatterton* v *Gerson* (1981), the judge, Bristow J., stated that, when the action is one of assault and battery, 'the consent must be real'. In expanding upon that statement, he said 'once the patient is informed in broad terms of the nature of the procedure which is intended, and gives her consent, that consent is real . . .'. He also recognised that the problem with this approach lies in its application.

It is possible to take the view that the *Chatterton* v *Gerson* test is satisfied very easily. In consequence, most people with learning disabilities are competent to consent to most forms of treatment. It is, however, extremely unclear as a test to apply in practice. Consequently, the Working Party convened by MENCAP on the Medical, Ethical and Issues of Mental Handicap considered what more specific guidance could be provided to determine the issue of competency. They concluded in their report, entitled *Competency and Consent to Medical Treatment*, that 'capacity is made up of five elements', which were then enumerated (MENCAP 1989). The Mental Health Act Code of Practice developed those elements and stated:

An individual in order to have capacity must be able to:

— understand what medical treatment is and that somebody has said that he needs it and why the treatment is being proposed;

— understand in broad terms the nature of the proposed treatment;
— understand its principal benefits and risks;
— understand what will be the consequences of not receiving the proposed treatment;
— possess the capacity to make a choice.

(Mental Health Act Code of Practice (1991), para. 15.15)

It is open to question whether this development of the test established in *Chatterton* v *Gerson* (1981) is a correct one. It is possible to argue that the approach propounded in the Code sets a higher standard for competency than does the 'real consent/broad terms' approach. If it is the case that there is a difference, and it is not clear that there is such a difference, it might be that the approach in the Code is to be regarded as the better approach. The Code attempts to assess what are the basic abilities that a person should have to be able to consent to treatment. It is not the case that the Code is setting a particularly high standard, but that it is saying that consent to treatment is not satisfied by merely understanding a rough explanation of what the treatment itself involves, and no consideration at all of, for example, alternative forms of treatment.

What is quite clear is that incompetency cannot be established on the basis of a label which a particular person carries. This is because the question of consent to treatment is concerned with a particular form of treatment at a particular time and is, therefore, very much an individualised and specific issue (Gunn 1987).

If a person is competent to consent to treatment, the issue may well arise as to how much information should be provided, that is where the issue of what is colloquially known as 'informed consent' arises. It will be noticed that this issue arises once the question of competence has been addressed. It arises under the heading of negligence and is, therefore, strictly of no direct relevance, because the law will be the same for a person with learning disabilities as for anyone else once it has been accepted that she or he is competent to decide.

If a person is thought not to be competent, it has to be considered whether the treatment can be provided. As a matter of law, it must be established whether there is any defence, other than consent, which is not available because of lack of capacity, and which may permit the bodily interference inherent in the provision of treatment. Until recently there was considerable argument about what the answer might be (Skegg 1974; Gunn 1987), but the House of Lords has now provided an answer. In the case of *Re F* (1989) the House was faced with needing to consider whether an adult woman who could not consent could be sterilised. It should be noted that the question of her competency was not addressed and the case gives no guidance as to that matter. The case relies upon the unchallenged professional assumption that the woman in question was not competent to consent to sterilisation or a form of contraception which would have avoided the need to consider sterilisation.

The House of Lords in *Re F* (1989) decided that the courts are not competent to create a structure within which decisions could be made on behalf of an incompetent adult. They do not have the same power over incompetent adults that they have over children to decide what is best. The approach that the House took was to recognise that the form of treatment in question involved bodily contact which would amount to an assault and battery unless the treatment provider had a defence. The only defence that the House recognised as being relevant was that of necessity.

The problem then was to consider how it is to be ascertained whether a particular treatment proposal was necessary. To this end the House proposed a two part test:

1. Is the treatment for the patient's life, health or wellbeing?
2. Is the treatment in the patient's best interests?

If the answer to both questions is yes, the treatment can be given because the defence of necessity is satisfied and so no assault or battery is committed when the treatment is carried out. If the answer is no to either question, the treatment cannot be given.

The first question means that treatment which is non-therapeutic may be covered by the defence of necessity and thus given to a person with learning disabilities. This follows from the addition of the phrase 'wellbeing', which is clearly intended to cover non-therapeutic sterilisation, which is what was proposed in the case itself. In consequence, cosmetic surgery and organ donation by the incompetent person to another may be permissible in some presumably very rare cases. In Canada, the Supreme Court, in exercising its own jurisdiction to decide what treatment can and cannot be provided to an incompetent adult, has decided that it is not entitled to authorise non-therapeutic treatment (*Re Eve* (1986)). The Supreme Court indicated that if non-therapeutic treatment were desirable, it was a matter for the legislature to debate and provide full guidelines upon.

The second question is also controversial. It is to be hoped that if the person in question has at some time indicated a treatment preference full account should be taken of it when assessing the appropriateness of a form of treatment. In Lord Goff's speech in *Re*

F there is an indication that account should be taken of such expressions of preference. This may suggest that, if possible, a substituted judgment test should be used rather than a best interests test. A substituted judgment test would have arrived at no different conclusion upon the presumed facts of the case, because there was no indication from the woman in question of what her decision would have been had she been competent to decide for herself. It can be seen though that if there ever was such information then a substituted judgment test could arrive at a significantly different decision which would enhance the propriety of giving respect to autonomy and self-determination rather than paternalism. For example, if a Jehovah's Witness has made clear his or her religious beliefs a further treatment decision would have to take those religious beliefs into account on a substituted judgment test, but not on a best interests test (*Malette* v *Shulman* (1990)).

Even greater controversy has been created by the way in which the House indicated that 'best interests' should be established. The House adopted the same test as appears in the law of negligence. So a form of treatment is in a patient's best interests if a responsible body of medical opinion would approve of the provision of that form of treatment to the patient in question. Unquestionably, this approach over-professionalises the matter. It leaves the decisions on treatment in the hands of the people exercising the same professional practice as the person proposing the treatment in question. It requires no consultation with other people, for example, carers, people from different professions and ethicists. It does not seem proper to equate that which is necessary with what is in a person's best interests. If sterilisation is in a person's best interests, will it follow automatically that it is necessary? Best interests could involve considerations outside the person in terms of her or his relationships, lifestyle, etc. An interference can only be necessary if it is required to preserve health or, probably, prevent serious damage to health (see, further, Morgan 1990). On the other hand, it would have been very difficult for the courts to have come up with a better approach which would have provided some form of guidance to practitioners. What is required, therefore, is some form of more detailed and careful consideration of the whole matter.

The difficulty of deciding when a proposed treatment is in the interests of a person who cannot indicate her or his own decision was faced by the MENCAP Working Party, which wished to encourage the creation of guidelines on a national basis as to the appropriate issues to take into account when considering specific forms of treatment, and the weight such factors should be given. As an example it indicated the sort of criteria which should be taken into account when the proposed treatment is sterilisation (MENCAP 1989).

Under the *Re F* (1989) approach, it is not for the court to decide upon these issues; the decision must be that of the treatment provider. He or she cannot be required to consult with anyone else, but the House of Lords indicated that it was good practice to do so. The House also indicated that a court declaration should be considered whenever the treatment proposal involved sterilisation. This cannot be required as a matter of law on the basis of the House's approach, because the only person who needs to assess the legality of her or his actions is the treatment provider, who needs a defence to what would otherwise be an assault and battery. However, the court may assist in that process by offering its opinion upon the legality of a proposed treatment through the issuing of a declaration one way or the other. Presumably, a court declaration is to be required in sterilisation cases because the form of treatment is not one which relies solely upon the assessment of medical criteria. If the sterilisation were proposed to cure cancer of the womb, the treatment might be easily approved and indeed there might be no need to go to court to seek the declaration (*J* v *C* (1990); *Official Solicitor's Practice Note* (1990)). Sterilisation is not the only form of treatment which involves significant non-medical questions. Other treatments of such a nature include cosmetic surgery, organ donations and terminations of pregnancy.

Surprisingly, a court has indicated that if a treatment provider is con-templating a termination of pregnancy and the criteria of the Abortion Act 1967 (as amended by the Human Fertilisation and Embryology Act 1990) are satisfied, there is no need to seek a court declaration (*Re SG* (1991)). This is an alarming approach. It serves to indicate some of the problems associated with resolving the problem of incapacity and consent. No-one not alleged to be incompetent would ever decide to have an abortion merely because the criteria of the 1967 Act were satisfied; why should the position be different for a person who cannot consent? There is nothing in *Re F* (1989) which suggests that this is a proper approach. It should be overruled and consigned to history.

The approach adopted in *Re F* would, therefore, appear to be flawed. At least reform of treatment decisions affecting people who are not competent to consent must be achieved. However, the problem of decision-making, incapacity and consent cannot be confined to treatment as the brief survey which follows of some of the legal issues which may arise in relation to an incompetent adult with learning disabilities will show.

MARRIAGE

Consent lies at the heart of marriage as a legal construct. Prior to the Nullity of Marriage Act 1971, if the consent of both parties was not present, a marriage was void. To describe a marriage as void means, amongst other things, that no valid marriage ever existed, despite the parties going through a ceremony, and that a decree ending the marriage is not required since no marriage exists (Cretney and Masson 1990: 31–3). However, since 31 July 1971 marriages are voidable where one or more of the parties did not validly consent to the marriage. The consequence of a marriage being said to be voidable is that it is regarded as a valid marriage until and unless someone obtains a decree to end it (Cretney and Masson 1990: 31–3). As the leading textbook puts the issue,

> Marriage . . . is a very simple contract, which it does not require a high degree of intelligence to understand. Mental illness or deficiency will only affect the validity of consent if either spouse was, at the time of the ceremony, by reason of the illness or deficiency, incapable of understanding the nature of marriage and the duties and responsibilities it creates.
>
> (Cretney and Masson 1990: 56; see also Whitehorn 1985)

Thus if a person with learning disabilities can go through the marriage ceremony, there will not be a void marriage, but it may be voidable. The issue of capacity to consent will usually, if at all, arise after the marriage and then only if someone seeks to have the marriage avoided. Ordinarily speaking only a party to the marriage may seek to obtain a decree to have the marriage ended through this procedure (Cretney and Masson 1990: 33). However, if the management of the property and affairs of a person with learning disabilities is under the control of the Court of Protection, that Court has jurisdiction to engage in legal proceedings involving the 'patient' (Mental Health Act 1983, s. 96 (1) (i)), including petitions on behalf of the patient for nullity of marriage and divorce (Whitehorn 1985: 241).

It is, in fact, possible to raise the question of capacity to consent to marriage before the ceremony in one of two ways: by dissent from the publication of banns and by way of entering a 'caveat'. The former is well known, the latter demands further consideration. Caveats may be entered with regard to both Church of England and other marriages. Church of England marriages are usually preceded by the reading out of banns, but in those rare cases where either a special licence or common licence is to be used, preliminary inquiries leading to the possible entering of a caveat may be made to the Bishop's

Registrar (Whitehorn 1985: 238). With marriages taking place after the issuing of a licence from the Superintendent Registrar, a caveat may be entered with that Registrar. Anyone may enter a caveat (Marriage Act 1949, s. 29(1)). Once it is entered, no certificate or licence may be issued by a Superintendent Registrar unless he or she has examined the matter and 'is satisfied that [the caveat] ought not to obstruct the issue of the certificate or licence . . .' (Marriage Act 1949, s. 29(2)). If the Registrar does not issue a licence or certificate, an appeal lies to the Registrar General (Marriage Act 1949, s. 29(3)).

The entering of a caveat may, therefore, raise the question of whether a person is competent to marry. That issue must be investigated if a caveat is entered, and so the marriage of a person or couple with learning disabilities may be made more difficult. It should be noted that no caveat is entered into lightly, since if it is, the expenses of any investigation fall upon the person who did so enter that caveat.

One other way of ending a marriage without seeking divorce is to establish one of the other grounds making a marriage voidable, and then seek a decree avoiding the marriage. The most relevant ground is to allege that, at the time of the marriage, the person, though capable of consenting, was suffering from mental disorder of such a kind or to such an extent as to be unfitted for marriage (Matrimonial Causes Act 1973, s. 12(d)).

SEXUAL INTERCOURSE

It has been made clear that simply because a woman submits to sexual intercourse does not mean that she is consenting to it (*R* v *Day* (1841), *R* v *Olugboja* (1981)). If a woman is deceived as to the nature and quality of the act she will not have consented to it (*R* v *Flattery* (1877), *R* v *Williams* (1923)). If, however, a woman is merely deceived as to the identity of the person with whom she has sexual intercourse, she has still consented to it. This is one of the more controversial aspects of the law of rape. It means that there is no rape unless the man pretends to be her husband in which case section 1(2) of the Sexual Offences Act 1956 makes clear that the man then does commit rape, that is sexual intercourse with a woman without her consent.

A person with learning disabilities may, therefore, consent to sexual intercourse (*R* v *Howard* (1966)) or sexual activity involving what would otherwise be an indecent assault (*R* v *Kimber* (1983)). However, complexity is added by a group of provisions in the Sexual Offences

Act 1956 which mean that if the person with learning disabilities can be described as a 'defective' as defined in the 1956 Act she or he cannot in law provide consent, which means that the person having sex with her or him commits an offence which, although it may not be rape, may be having unlawful sexual intercourse with a woman who is a defective or indecently assaulting a man or a woman who is a defective (see Gunn 1991 for a fuller discussion).

REFORM

Decision-making by and for people who are incapable of deciding for themselves has given rise to such concern that the Law Commission has been asked to consider the whole of the law relating to decision-making and mentally incapacitated adults and, if necessary, make recommendations for change by legislation. The Commission has so far produced a consultation document entitled, *Mentally Incapacitated Adults and Decision-Making* (Law Commission 1991).

The survey of existing law by the Commission and the examples of the law considered above indicate that there is quite a considerable amount of law dealing with the issue, but that there are problems which need to be faced and resolved. One clear problem is that the law is fragmented. It is not to be found in one source, but in many different sources. The law that there is, is related solely to the making of particular decisions and consequently different answers and procedures apply. Thus, the issues of competency to consent to a particular treatment bear no necessary relationship to marriage or the management of property and affairs. Second, when the particular legal approaches are considered they can be seen to be often unclear and complex. This should be quite obvious from the complexity of the legal arguments indicated by the preceding discussion. Third, it can be seen that some of the answers provided by the law are simply unacceptable, the most obvious example being the one provided to the consent to treatment issue, where methods of arriving at a decision are not acceptable, especially when set against the values and principles outlined by the Law Commission and set out above.

Fourth, as the Law Commission points out, even where procedures do exist for assessing incompetency and determining what should be done if a person is found to be incompetent, they are often not used. There is often a desire amongst carers to use informal methods to resolve a matter, even if that resolution has a legally dubious basis. This approach is perhaps classically expressed in many people's desire to avoid using the Court of Protection to deal with matters relating to the management of an incapable person's property and affairs. The Court still has the reputation of being overly bureaucratic, slow, outdated and expensive, despite the considerable changes which have been effected under the present Master (Carson 1987). Fifth, account must be taken of the possible stigmatisation which may be associated with the use of the various legal procedures. The undesirability of stigmatisation may be another factor encouraging carers to use informal, legally questionable methods. Sixth, whilst informal approaches have their advantages in avoiding stigmatisation, involving appropriate parties and not being bureaucratic, 'patients are deprived of the procedural safeguards' that are contained in formal procedures and 'that, whilst it may work in the majority of cases in the context of a caring family supported by well motivated professionals, in a minority of cases it can make it easier for rogues to prey upon mentally incapacitated people with less chance of discovery or intervention' (Law Commission 1991: 100).

Finally, it must be doubted whether all decisions which an adult might make can be made on behalf of a person not capable of making such decisions for her or himself. An obvious example is that it is not clear who may decide where an incompetent adult is to live. If the management of her or his property and affairs have been brought under the control of the Court of Protection, its decisions as to how the money should be spent will be highly influential. However, it may often be the case that there is a dispute between carers and professionals over the most appropriate accommodation. There is no way of resolving such disputes unless formal powers under either the National Assistance Acts 1946 and 1951 or the Mental Health Act 1983 are used. These are formal procedures which all people involved have a natural reluctance to invoke for the reasons already considered. In any case they will frequently be irrelevant when the incompetent adult is a person with learning disabilities.

HOW MIGHT REFORM BE APPROACHED?

On the basis of the principles and values which the Law Commission identified, and which are enumerated above, it considered what is 'the best broad approach'. The Commission identified three possible approaches to reform:

1. 'The minimalist', that is 'a general "tidying up" exercise, aimed at removing the main anomalies and obstacles and encouraging a greater use of existing provisions without any wholesale revision of the law.'

2. 'The incremental', that is a separate examination of 'particular areas, or particular kinds of problem, with a view to up-dating, or if necessary thoroughly reforming, the law on that subject.'

3. 'The overall', that is 'a full long term investigation into all aspects of decision-making on behalf of mentally incapacitated adults with a view to recommending the creation of a comprehensive code of law and practice aimed at providing a solution, at an appropriate level, to all problems which are likely to arise.'

(Law Commission 1991: 97–9)

Bearing in mind those possible general approaches, the Law Commission indicated a number of 'options for change'. Some of them, such as introducing advance directives, are not of much concern to people with learning disabilities, because they require an ability to indicate in advance some treatment or other decision preference or to choose a decision-maker. If a person with learning disabilities is incompetent, this is unlikely to be a practical option. If a person with learning disabilities is competent, it may be relevant, but in the same way as for anyone else. Of greater interest are first the options which develop on existing procedures or, at least, do not indicate a wholesale change to current methods of approach, and, second, the option of introducing a completely new system.

Without introducing a completely new system, it would be possible to clarify and regularise or legalise current methods whereby decisions are made on behalf of an incompetent adult. So it would be possible to look to a representative already formally appointed such as a guardian or receiver, a responsible professional, the primary carer, the family, a combination of professional, primary carer and family, or a court, tribunal or other authority. It would also be possible to introduce substitute consent to treatment procedures. It was this approach which was put forward by the MENCAP Working Party. Their Report recommended the introduction of a scheme involving decisions usually being taken by relative and doctor, but any disputes between relative and doctor, any doubts raised by other interested parties and treatment proposals involving special treatments, such as sterilisation, being referred to a local committee for advice or guidance (within the current legal structure) or decision (if introduced via a new procedure). One further option was that of extended minority, however, whereas both these two options so far mentioned might, with the introduction of appropriate safeguards, satisfy the principle and values, it seems unlikely that this could be said of extended minority which carries the most obviously damaging possible consequence of infantilisation.

Further, it would be possible to improve existing procedures. Of the possibilities addressed, the Law Commission identified that it 'would be possible to devise a simple protective mechanism to allow intervention to protect a vulnerable adult from neglect or abuse' (Law Commission 1991: 160). One option considered by the Law Commission was that put forward by Age Concern recommending an Emergency Intervention Order (Age Concern 1986). Second, it would be possible to expand the scope of current guardianship procedures under the Mental Health Act 1983 at least to permit a treatment decision to be made, although this has its major drawbacks in terms of applicability in particular. Third, the role of the Court of Protection could be expanded. These options have the advantage of responding to particular identified problems and providing a specific response and consequently might be attractive as a relatively simple means of responding to the identified problem. However, these options do not seem adequately to address the problem presented by the inability of the mentally incapacitated adult and decision-making, although they do address specific issues. They offer no guarantee that all decisions can be made on behalf of an incompetent adult, they do nothing to solve the problems of fragmentation (if that is a significant problem), or complexity. Professionals and carers might well have as much difficulty as at present of knowing what avenues to use in order to respond appropriately to the needs of a person who cannot make her or his own decisions. There is a real chance that such procedures might not be used for similar reasons to those affecting current procedures. Finally, there is nothing in these options which does anything other than respond to a problem. They are not proactive nor concerned with developing the potential of a person with learning disabilities to act independently.

In consequence, the preferable option might be to seek to introduce a completely new system, although it involves a relatively formal procedure (see Carney and Singer 1986: ch. 8). Many countries have systems of guardianship, but not all are plenary in form. Plenary guardianship applies where a person is not competent to make any decisions and thus the guardian must make all decisions on her or his behalf. It is also recognised that many people are capable of making at least some decisions and so the more frequently used form of guardianship is limited guardianship to enable decisions, for example, with regard to some forms of treatment or the management of property and affairs to be made (see McLaughlin 1979; Carney and Singer 1986).

The Law Commission considered the experiences in Canada (see also McLaughlin 1979), Australia (see also Carney and Singer 1986), New Zealand, Scandinavia, Austria and Germany (see also Shaw 1990). From this survey the Commission concluded that there were a number of common threads running through the new legislation introduced or being introduced in these various countries:

> It tends to be focused on the rights, interests and welfare of the person concerned, and is aimed at enabling mentally incapacitated people to gain greater freedom and independence.
>
> (Law Commission 1991: 131)

A common thread is the use of some form of guardianship, that is the appointment of people, the guardians, who

> generally have two main responsibilities, exercising rights on behalf of the mentally incapacitated person or assisting him to exercise his own rights if this is possible, and protecting his interests. The legislation in different countries strives to find ways of balancing these reflections of the conflict between autonomy and paternalism.
>
> (Law Commission 1991: 132)

Most proposals do not permit guardianship unless 'the needs of the person cannot be met by other means' and then only permit the use of

> limited guardianship, which allows the extent of the guardian's authority to be tailored to the particular needs of the person concerned. Plenary orders are permitted only when they are strictly necessary and are rare.
>
> (Law Commission 1991: 133)

Further, the Commission noted that there

> is a growing trend towards legal and procedural safeguards against abuse or the undue restriction of rights. Safeguards adopted in different jurisdictions differ, but include combinations of the following:
>
> (i)   widely drawn standing to make an application;
> (ii)   improvement in the quality of hearings, some of which are held in public;
> (iii) provision for notice to be given to anyone likely to have a useful point of view to contribute;
> (iv)   a presumption that the person concerned will attend, often backed up by provision for him to be interviewed if he does not;
> (v)   representation for the person whose capacity is subject to challenge;

(vi)   provisions for more rigorous testing of medical evidence and for assessments of social competence;

(vii) power to obtain specialist reports;

(viii) prescribed time limits;

(ix)   regular reviews;

(x)   an appeal procedure;

(xi)   provision for reasoned decisions to be given.

There is a conflict between the need for 'due process', represented by procedural safeguards and standards of proof, and welfare considerations which suggest that proceedings should be easily accessible, inquisitorial and conducted in an informal atmosphere.

(Law Commission 1991: 134–5; and see Carney and Singer 1986)

Whichever option is pursued, it seems that it is essential that advocacy of some form is introduced. Clearly self-advocacy is of most value not only in enabling a person to make her or his own decisions, but also in emphasising the need to develop everyone's potential with the objective of achieving independence. There is nothing to stop the introduction of such schemes, but government encouragement and funding would enable much greater success to be achieved. However, in some cases self-advocacy may not be a practical option, in which case citizen advocacy is worthy of consideration. Whilst recognising all the problems, not least of which are funding and availability of people prepared to act as advocates, this approach has the advantage of providing an advocate who gets to know a person who cannot make her or his own decisions well and who is not professionally involved. Such a scheme could easily be introduced by the implementation of the Disabled Persons (Services, Consultation and Representation) Act 1986.

REFERENCES

Books, articles, etc.

Age Concern (1986) *The Law and Vulnerable Elderly People*. London: Age Concern.

Carney, T. and Singer, P. (1986) *Ethical and Legal Issues in Guardianship Options for Intellectually Disadvantaged People*. Canberra: Australian Government Publishing Service.

Carson, D. (ed.) (1987) *Making the Most of the Court of Protection*. London: King's Fund Centre.

Cretney, S.M. and Masson, J.M. (1990) *Principles of Family Law*. (5th edn) London: Sweet and Maxwell.

Fennell, P. (1990) 'Inscribing Paternalism in the Law: Consent to Treatment and Mental Disorder', *Journal of Law and Society*, 17, 29–51.

Gunn, M.J. (1987) 'Treatment and mental handicap', *Anglo-American Law Review*, 16, 242–67.

Gunn, M.J. (1991) *Sex and the Law: a brief guide for staff working with people with learning difficulties*. London: Family Planning Association.

Law Commission (1991) *Mentally Incapacitated Adults and Decision-Making: An Overview* (LC Consultation Paper No. 119), London: HMSO.

McLaughlin, P. (1979) *Guardianship of the Person*. Ontario: NIMR.

MENCAP (1989) *Competency and Consent to Medical Treatment*, report of the working party on the legal, medical and ethical issues of mental handicap. London: MENCAP.

Mental Health Act Code of Practice (1991) London: HMSO.

Morgan, D. (1990) 'Commentary on Re F'. *Journal of Social Welfare Law*, 204–7.

Official Solicitor's Practice Note (1990) 2 F.L.R. 530.

Shaw, J. (1990) 'Sterilization of Mentally Handicapped People: Judges Rule OK?' *Modern Law Review*, 53, 91–106.

Skegg, P.D.G. (1974) 'A justification for medical procedures performed without consent'. *Law Quarterly Review*, 90, 512–30.

United Nations (1971) *Declaration of the Rights of Mentally Retarded Persons*. New York: UN Dept of Social Affairs.

Whitehorn, N. (1985) *Heywood and Massey's Court of Protection Practice*. London: Steven and Sons.

Cases

Chatterton v *Gerson* (1981) Law Reports: Queens Bench 432

Collins v *Wilcock* (1984) 3 All England Law Reports 374

Re Craig (1971) Law Reports: Chancery 95

Re Eve (1986) 31 Dominion Law Reports 4th series 1

Re F (1989) 1 All England Law Reports 545

Freeman v *Home Office* (1984) 1 All England Law Reports 1036

J v *C* (1990) 1 Weekly Law Reports 1248

R v *Blaue* (1975) 1 Weekly Law Reports 1411

R v *Day* (1841) 9 Carrington and Payne Reports 722

R v *Flattery* (1877) 2 Queens Bench Division Reports 410

R v *Howard* (1966) 1 Weekly Law Reports 13

R v *Kimber* (1983) 1 Weekly Law Reports 1118

R v *Olugboja* (1981) 73 Criminal Appeal Reports 344

R v *Williams* (1923) 1 Law Reports: Kings Bench 340

Re SG (1991) *The Times*, 31 January

Mallete v *Shulman* (1990) 67 Dominion Law Reports (4th series) 321 (Canada)

Schloendorff v *Society of New York Hospitals* (1914) 105 North Eastern Reports 92

T v *T* (1988) 1 All England Law Reports 613

Wellesley v *Vere* (1841) 2 Curteis' Reports 917

Wilson v *Pringle* (1986) 2 All England Law Reports 440

7 Between ourselves

Experiences of a women's group on sexuality and sexual abuse

Lorraine Millard

INTRODUCTION

I was asked to contribute a chapter to this book following the release of the video *Between Ourselves* (Twentieth Century Vixen 1988). The video is about a women's group I co-ran for women with moderate learning disabilities. It shows some of the women and myself talking about a number of the issues that arise in the group and demonstrates some of the methods we used to explore them.

In common with many women's groups it allowed safe and confidential space to look at: feelings, life experience and sexuality. The group was not set up as a survivors' group and I certainly did not enter it as a group leader with any expertise in the area of sexual abuse and learning disability. However, what emerged very soon was that several of the women had been and were being sexually assaulted. My co-worker and I were very clear that we were not going to deny or silence the issue further, so, together with the group, we found ways to work with it.

After eighteen months of working together we all felt we wanted to document our experience and put it to positive use. We wanted to campaign for the rights of all women with learning disabilities to have access to a women's group. With this same motivation we agreed to contribute to this chapter.

We had chosen to make a video for two reasons: because we felt it was the best way to communicate with other women in a similar position and because it was the only medium which would represent the women talking for themselves. As one of the women put it:

> It's important to say something you can see. To see things that you have made to show that you have tried. . . . It's good to have something that comes from our own mouths without anybody telling us what to say.

As for the writing of this chapter, few of the women had any literacy skills, so writing certainly did not give them the freedom to speak for themselves. Furthermore, our group has closed and I and my co-leader have left the agency. Due to other commitments my co-leader decided she could not participate in the writing. I felt it would be unfair and disruptive to both the women and the worker who had replaced me, to set up the group again simply for the purpose of compiling the chapter. With a mutual desire to give the project 'a go' we all agreed that I would meet members individually and, with their permission, tape them talking about the group. After transcribing the script it was obvious that the written medium would not do justice to them or their experiences. I did not want to direct, interpret or change their words in order to make them readable. This would have been dishonest and amounts again to putting words into their mouths. At their suggestion it was decided that I would write the chapter from my own perspective, but about our experience, and I would include quotes from them.

The chapter will look at: how and why we set up the group, how the issue of sexual abuse arose, some of the ways we found to work with the feelings engendered and how and why we went on to make the video.

BACKGROUND INFORMATION

> We want a group with no men to talk about our bodies, our problems and having babies.

In May 1986 I started work at Islington Elfrida Rathbone. Elfrida Rathbone is an agency that aims to meet the various needs of people with moderate learning disabilities. In Islington the organisation provides a range of services including the recreation unit where I was based. It is primarily a group work unit specialising in creative and therapeutic work. Individuals attend the unit on a voluntary basis and choose groups which are of interest to them.

I had been employed specifically as a woman worker alongside two male colleagues. It soon became apparent that the women in the unit had missed the presence of a woman worker and had very clear ideas of what they wanted from me. One of the most assertive and verbal women was the first to approach me to ask for a group just for women. Consequently I set up a meeting with them to discuss it further and we established that they wanted a closed, confidential group to talk about women's issues and to include sex education and standing up for themselves. My next task was to set up the group and find a co-worker.

My first instinct was to hold the group in a local women's centre. This would have introduced the women to a resource that was not solely for people with learning disabilities but was identified with women in general. Unfortunately, this proved impossible to achieve. The only suitable venues we could find were too difficult to travel to and would have required additional transport. As the recreation unit was familiar to women we decided to stay there. We timed it between 4 p.m. and 6 p.m. because this was late enough to allow women who had children to collect them from school, or to complete their day-time classes or work, but was early enough to make sure they could get home again safely.

Finding a co-worker was the next step. This proved very easy. The agency's Literacy Unit had already made provision to run a women-only class led by Nikki Seargent. Nikki and I agreed to combine the two projects. The women involved were familiar with Nikki and very happy to have her as one of the leaders.

PHILOSOPHY

We want to learn how to have rights.

Nikki and I had both experienced empowerment and clarity from having access to women's groups and the politics and literature generated by the women's movement. We had benefited from having somewhere to share our experiences and to set them within a political context rather than as isolated, individual problems. We saw this group as being no different to any other women's group except that having a learning disability compounded the feelings of a negative identity.

Women's groups are usually confidential groups where participants have the means to gain control over our memories and experiences without the fear of others taking control or acting on disclosures. Having a learning disability meant for most of the women that others always had control and power in their lives and they had little choice over where and with whom they chose to speak. Nor did they have the economic freedom to seek therapeutic or counselling help. It was enormously important that the women within the group should have this control and right to confidentiality respected. It was necessary to make it clear to social workers and, where appropriate, carers that this was the case before the start of the group, because groups for people with learning disabilities over the age of eighteen often are given no confidentiality. At this point we had not anticipated that the group would be dealing with disclosures of sexual abuse. When this happened we actively supported and empowered women to tell their social workers. We were never compromised in our promise of confidentiality due to fear for the women's safety.

AIMS OF THE GROUP

— To provide a safe, trusting and confidential environment in which the women felt confident enough to express themselves, no matter what problems they had in articulating.
— To be an empowering experience[1] which would give the women confidence and help them gain some control over their lives – develop assertiveness and decision-making skills.
— To develop relationships with each other.
— To enable them to find ways to express their feelings and share them with each other.
— To provide sex education.
— To make accessible general information re women's lives, women's health and sexual politics.
— To enable them to put their lives and experiences within the context of all women in our society. To help them identify with women in general and benefit from the progress achieved by the women's movement.
— To make them feel valued and listened to.
— To give them space to share their experience of having a learning disability.
— To have fun and enjoy themselves.

OBJECTIVES

We felt that empowerment and assertiveness could not be gained from isolated one-off sessions but had to be engendered through the culture of the group. We felt they had to be inherent throughout the group process and built into its structure by awareness, respect and sharing of power.

In keeping with this we did not prepare a set curriculum but planned each week as the group progressed so that we were directed by their needs and requests. The group then had control over the boundaries and content of discussions and activities.

CRITERIA FOR JOINING THE GROUP

We already had a core group of five women but felt we had room to invite other women, up to a maximum of ten. Although we felt there would be some problems integrating newcomers into a group who already knew each other we felt the benefits outweighed the difficulties. The core group was eager to expand and we discussed with them the importance of being open and sharing with new members. Any woman between the ages of eighteen and fifty who had a moderate learning difficulty was invited to meet with myself and Nikki. From these women we had to work out who could respect the issue of confidentiality since this was an essential requirement set by the women. This was difficult and included the painful task of turning women away who obviously needed a women's group but were unable to meet this criterion.

STRUCTURE OF THE GROUP

Very early on we decided that this would be a close rather than open group. This meant that it had a fixed membership and that women made a commitment to attend regularly. In all the group ran for a period of two years.

THE GROUP MEMBERS

We had an overall membership of nine women. Four self-referred from the recreation unit. Three were referred to us from other parts of the agency. The two women who joined us later were referred from a social worker and a counselling agency.

By their own definition, two were black British, one Nigerian, four white British and two Irish. Their ages ranged from eighteen to thirty-eight. All were identified as having moderate learning difficulties and had attended a special school. All of the women communicated verbally with widely differing levels of articulation, one woman had English as a second language. All of the women experienced problems with literacy. One woman had a child living with her, another had a child temporarily living in care. As the group progressed one woman clearly identified herself as a lesbian. Four lived with parents, three in their own accommodation, three lived in hostels/sheltered accommodation. Initially five women had social workers, and we arranged for two more to be allocated with social workers as circumstances necessitated it and at their request.

Two left after three months, as they had received full-time employment and felt they could no longer make a commitment to the group. I would like to acknowledge how much they contributed to the group in its vital early stage.

THE FIRST MEETING

Aims

This was set up as a social occasion with tea and biscuits. The aim of this meeting was to give the women an opportunity to make an informed choice about whether the group was right for them before making a commitment to membership. We used this session to make a list of expectations and ground rules and give them the space to ask us questions.

Plan

Whilst having tea and biscuits we introduced the idea of each woman having a bit of space for herself at the beginning of each session (we included ourselves in this). For this first session we used it for general introductions and to add something we liked doing. It was stressed that it was important that we were each listened to and respected during this time, including our right to remain silent if we so wished. This ritual remained with us throughout the two years, but changed to something good and bad that had happened to us during the week. At first some women were reluctant to use this space. However, in time they all used it and came to relish it, carefully guarding their own and each other's time. In fact, they asked for it to be extended as the weeks progressed.

To focus the group on women's issues and elicit information from them as to what was important in their lives, we drew two big pictures of women and labelled them:

1 Things which are important to women.
2 What things cause women problems?

As in initial stages of any group, participation varied. We encouraged the women to take some control and recognised their differing ways of contribution in getting them to draw the pictures and where possible do the writing. After filling in these pictures we made a list of the things they wanted to include in the group discussions. These were:

our bodies
sex
having babies
contraception
jobs
men and relationships
standing up for our rights
going out and having fun
going to a special school
feeling angry and depressed
moving away from home
cooking
going out as a group together
money
having fun.

Ground rules

Following this we asked them to make a list of rules they wanted in the group. I think it would be misleading simply to present the list so where necessary I will go into some detail as to why rules were chosen and how they were implemented.

1   Keeping stuff to ourselves

We discussed the issue of confidentiality in some detail and what it meant. As most of them had never been in a confidential group before they were very anxious to make sure it was respected and wanted to know what would be done if someone broke the rule. Together they decided that if it happened once it would be talked about to see if it was a mistake, if it happened more than once the woman would be asked to leave unless there was a good excuse. We never had to act on this but did have to clarify the boundaries around confidentiality at times as it did cause some confusion relating to:

a Respecting women's individual boundaries   Women did not have to talk about personal things. It was their right to keep boundaries around what they shared and they should not be automatically expected to trust the group. This was particularly important for the women that had outside connections with each other and each other's families and friends. One woman chose never to share her disclosure of abuse with the whole group. She told me about what had been evoked for her after the group and I helped her to set up individual counselling sessions with her social worker.

b   Appropriate boundaries outside of the group   We acknowledged that things might come up for them which could not be contained simply within the group and that it was fine for them to talk about these things in private with other people. Choosing appropriate people and places to take issues was a difficult concept for the women to understand so we illustrated it by the use of a sculpting exercise.

Each woman was given a large sheet of paper and a range of objects. Placing an object to represent themselves in the middle of the paper they arranged other people in their lives and the places they went to around them. Then each woman was given time within the group to work out where, when and with whom it was appropriate to share the various issues that came up for her in her life. We affirmed that it was never appropriate to talk about another woman's personal experience outside.

2   No interrupting each other

We decided that the group had to take collective responsibility for this and devised a signal – putting up and moving a hand to stop if it happened. The same applied if more than one person talked at a time.

3   No hitting

4   No shouting at each other

5   No running out

The women wanted this rule because in the past they had found that someone running out meant that the group leaders were taken away from them and the whole group was unfairly disrupted. They decided that if a woman was upset or needed time out for any other good reason this was fine so long as it was explained. Where appropriate it was also OK for one of us or a friend from the group to go with her. But absolutely no running out of the building.

6   No putting a woman down because of the way they looked or spoke, or because of their colour or disability. In time this extended to sexuality.

7 No turning up very late unless there was a good excuse.

8 No missing more than two sessions unless there was a good excuse and where possible letting us know if they could not turn up.

9 No gossiping about someone if they were not there.

10 Taking turns at making tea and washing up.

11 No swearing. This rule was later dropped because women needed to swear if they were angry or upset.

12 No men in the room at any time, not even workers.

We then had more tea and finalised arrangements for coming the following week. All the women decided that they wanted to continue with the group and agreed to make a commitment to it.

EARLY DAYS – THE FORMING

It took a few weeks for the group to settle into its first phase. Given the problem women with learning disabilities have attending groups we did not close the membership until the fourth week. By this time the women had had a chance to get to know us and each other and to feel comfortable with the structure. We had employed a number of activities to elicit things which they liked/did not like about themselves and their lives and had used drawing, masks and drama to look at how they expressed their feelings. By the fourth week they were eager to start with our agenda and priorities: looking at our bodies, to be followed by sex education and having babies.

OUR BODIES

It is embarrassing talking about our bodies, but it's important and they are ours, we need to know about how they work and names.

We did not use ready-made pictures or material for this because we wanted to start from where the group was at. We needed to ascertain what they knew and the words they used to name body parts. Further, the drawings we had available were very basic and exclusively of slim, white, able-bodied women which did not reflect the women in the group.

Again, we employed the help of big pictures of women, but this time we asked for volunteers who felt comfortable lying down and being drawn around. It is important to be sensitive with this exercise. Lying down is a very vulnerable position and having other people do things around your body can evoke frightening and painful memories for any woman who has been sexually abused in this way. It can also be a negative experience for anyone who feels uncomfortable with their body image or shape.

Using the outlines of the women's bodies we drew and labelled all the parts they could identify. It started easily enough including features like eyes, legs, brain, but teetered to silence and giggles when we reached the sexual parts of a woman's body. It was not only embarrassment which halted our progress, it was lack of vocabulary and knowledge. The only words they did know to describe the vagina or breasts were words they felt uncomfortable using. In response we devised a game to help us use words that we found difficult. Using a ball we threw it to each other, each time a woman received the ball she named a body part. This greatly relaxed the atmosphere and created a sense of fun and control. The women enjoyed this game and so we used it for several weeks. At first it was Nikki and I that said the difficult words but over time the women were saying them for themselves. Every time a new word came up it was explained and added to the picture. With confidence the women shared all the names they used for the sexual parts of their bodies, including those they found painful, like 'cunt'. Saying the words and having some control over them both defused their abusive potential and helped them re-own these parts for themselves. Working at the women's pace it took several weeks to have a complete picture of the women's body but the process ensured that the information was clearly shared.

Identifying body parts was one thing, owning and dealing with how the women felt about their body parts, particularly those to do with sexuality, quite another. An additional picture of a woman was created, this time to look at the feelings we have. This woman developed a character of her own. They named her Elfrida, dressed her, aged her twenty-five; they said she had a learning disability and talked about how this affected her life. Through Elfrida the women could talk about their bodies and their feelings in a safe, distanced way. Thus we would ask, 'How does she feel about her body?', 'How does she feel when she hears a woman being called a slag?', 'Does she ever feel sexy?', 'Does having a learning disability make her feel different to other women?' With the help of Elfrida we were able to openly clarify that the women felt a sense of shame about their bodies, they felt the sexual parts of them were dirty and unpleasant.

Nikki and I used this opportunity to put their lives in a political and social context. We talked about the images of women in society, about pornography and the ways they had traditionally been put down and made to feel ashamed of their bodies and their sexuality. We also opened the subject of violence against women and sexual abuse. We played the ball game, this time using the words that hurt and abused them and they became angry with the fact that we could find no equivalent words for 'slag' or 'slut' which applied to men.

This proved extremely empowering for the women and their anger and sense of injustice fired them to make a poster for the Rec. It read:

> Words like slag, tart, slut or whore are banned from the Rec. They are sexist and any man who uses them or puts us down because of our body will be asked to leave. We feel good about our bodies and won't be put down anymore.

The women were now ready to move away from Elfrida and talk for themselves. They were eager for more information. They wanted to know about women's body processes, and to take a closer look at the vagina. We used a menstrual calendar to explore the first. Each woman was given a chart to monitor her monthly cycle. Through subsequent discussions the women realised that swollen breasts, mood swings, vaginal discharges, etc. were both 'normal' and common occurrences for women. This enabled them to talk about their own bodies much more openly.

Collectively we made a large clay model of a woman to look at the vagina. We wanted to put it within the context of the whole woman and found isolated pictures or photographs of the vagina inappropriate. The model included all of the woman's body and we had great fun when it came to the genitals: putting the anus in the right place, debating the size of the labia and ceremoniously placing the clitoris. In the context of a relaxed and humorous activity the group were able to explore what was sexually pleasing for women and own the vagina for themselves.

GENERAL SEX EDUCATION

Most women don't enjoy sex, we're just being used.

The women in the group had no sense of their own sexuality and no belief that they could have, had the right to, sexual pleasure. It is a myth to say that they had no sex education: from the world around them they had taken in sexist and damaging messages about their bodies and sex, but nothing about their sexuality and choice.

Knowing that women can and do enjoy sex must be a prerequisite to sex education in general. We affirmed with the group that it was their right only to engage in sex with another person if they felt emotionally and physically ready for it, that it was fine to have sex with either a man or a woman if they felt good about it and that they had the right to stop what was happening at any point if they did not like or want it.

We engaged the help of a sex education agency to work on this issue. We were extremely fortunate to have a woman worker who both shared our philosophy towards the work and had previous experience of working with women with learning disabilities. We agreed that she would use the material she had in a women-orientated way. Most of the sex education material we had previously seen focused on men, preparation for sex being a kiss, the signal to go further an erect penis followed by penetration. We clearly wanted to avoid colluding with this message. She also agreed to cover different kinds of relationships, contraception, possible pregnancy and the choices around that. Initially she was to come for three weeks, but due to the necessary slow pace and the issues that arose she remained with us for eight weeks in all.

On the second week she showed some pictures and slides. The women's response to these, specifically those of naked men and the man's penis, was telling. We had expected embarrassment and giggles; we got those, but also clear distress. Recognising this, it was obviously not appropriate to continue, so we stopped and gave time to talk about what had happened. It was a difficult discussion. Some felt fine about the pictures and could talk easily, but all were affected by the obvious silence of other members. The feeling of tension was overwhelming. It was apparent that we needed to re-evaluate the process and give the control back to the women. The women concluded that although they wanted to continue with the sex education they did not want it every week. They agreed to have it fortnightly with the alternative weeks spent on a relaxing, easier activity. We were lucky that our colleague, Gail, was able and prepared to fit in with this. We also agreed that the three of us would stay around for half an hour after the group so that if any woman wanted to she could talk to one of us in private. None of the women took us up on this.

SEXUAL ABUSE

After the group Nikki, Gail and myself spent considerable time trying to work out what was going on. With the supportive guidance and experience of Gail we were able to recognise that we were dealing with the issue of sexual abuse. In retrospect, given the nature and content of the group, and my subsequent knowledge of how common sexual abuse is for women with learning disabilities, it is only surprising that it did not come up earlier. I can only conclude that neither we as group leaders, nor the women, were ready to recognise or work with it before. One of the common strengths in women who have been sexually abused is that they are very attuned to other people's feelings and reactions. Having also been actively silenced, they have needed to protect themselves emotionally and physically from inappropriate or potentially dangerous disclosures. In my experience this is no different for women with moderate learning disabilities. The women in the group who had been abused were waiting for a signal from us that we were able to hear and believe them. We felt it was vital to honour the woman's right to choose her time and means of telling. We feared that the pictures may have provoked associations that were unbidden and therefore out of the women's control. We needed to acknowledge that something had come up whilst containing the process. Containing it so that the women could regain control and so that we could prepare ourselves and be ready and able to hear.

Wisely the women had provided us with the primary means of containment with their suggestion of fortnightly sessions. Respecting their wishes we planned to take their lead in the following week, giving them space to work on the activity of their choice. Gail would return as arranged, but without the slides, and would generally slow down the sex education process. We agreed to keep the private time option open, following each sex education session. In the subsequent weeks some women did use it. It was during these private sessions that we had our first disclosures of abuse. These women were not ready to share their experiences with the group so with their agreement we worked with them to get outside support.

HOW SEXUAL ABUSE CAME OPENLY INTO THE GROUP

The next week all the women turned up for the group. They all appeared fine and nothing alluding to the previous week came up in the ritual opening. We broached the subject and they assertively reiterated that they wanted space away from it. They said that they were happy to return to it the following week but wanted something completely different from this session. They chose a drama project, saying they wanted to work on a play to span the alternative weeks of the sex education. The play went as follows:

Session I

A group of women living together in a house with one man. For reasons not given the man upset them and very angrily and assertively they made him leave. They then rearranged the house and chose new rooms for themselves and decorated them in the styles and colours of their choosing.

Session II

They worked out how they were going to survive and keep themselves. They went to the DHSS to get some money. They became very angry with the way they were treated at the DHSS and acted out telling the workers exactly what they thought of them. Their anger was fired by having to fill out so many forms when they could not read nor write. They assertively demanded help adding that having a learning disability did not mean they were stupid and that they wanted to be treated with respect.

Session III

They decided that some of them needed to go out to work, they looked at the different skills they had and went off to various job interviews. They got the jobs. One of them was touched up by a man at work. We identified this as sexual harassment so they took him to court and won.

Session IV

Relaxing in their beautiful home with lots of money they arranged a party for themselves. At the party they looked back over what had happened and why they got rid of the man who had originally lived in the house (see Session I). It came out that some of the women had been hit and sexually abused by him. With our intervention they decided he too should go to court, that what had happened was very wrong and that in no way could it have been their fault.

The issue of sexual abuse had been openly discussed. After the session we talked more about it, reiterating that they were in no way to blame and adding that it happened to lots of women. Two of the women talked about what had happened to them. It is important to state that not all the women had been sexually abused but they all shared being verbally abused and felt both angry and upset about it.

Both of these disclosures were about past abuses which the women did not want to do anything about, they just wanted to talk and be heard.

After this they no longer wanted the play or alternative activity weeks. The play had provided the same function as Elfrida: through it they were able to distance themselves and feel safe enough to express their opinions and feelings. It also provided them with the means to rehearse talking and test out reactions. It gave them a contained outlet for a range of feelings, primarily anger. It helped them to explore their survival techniques, their skills and assertiveness.

Unbeknownst to all of us the women themselves created the circumstances which enabled them to bring sexual abuse openly in the group. I learnt two important lessons from this: first, the importance of giving women control of the process; second, trusting that, given the right circumstances, women who have been sexually abused will find a way to express it when the time is right.

WAYS OF WORKING WITH SEXUAL ABUSE

> I think people with learning difficulties should have a campaign about being sexually abused and there should be more women's groups for lesbians.

> There are centres for rape crises . . . not much use if you haven't got a phone . . . but at least they don't just tell you to go away . . . .

I wish to reiterate here that the group was not set up as a survivors' group, nor did it become one. It was a women's group which, as I stated earlier, aimed to take direction from the women and work with whatever issues came up for them. Sexual abuse is a reality in women's lives and was certainly a major issue for several of the women in the group. Being determined not to silence these women further we did our utmost to acknowledge it and ensure that the group was a safe place for them to share their experiences and work through them.

Following the disclosures described above, sexual abuse did become the focus of the group for a while. It was compounded by the fact that one of the members was raped during this time. She chose to bring her experience to the group first. With the very sensitive help and support of the other women she was able to find a voice to talk about what had happened and her pain. The group empowered her by consistent endorsement that:

— it was not her fault
— she was not to blame

— it happened to lots of women and therefore not because of anything particular about her
— she was valuable and deserved justice and protection.

This in turn enabled her to tell her social worker and report it to the police.

Holding the feelings

This incident profoundly affected the whole group, especially those who had been sexually abused. We needed to find a way to contain yet allow expression of a whole range of feelings and emotions like: rage, fear, sadness, powerlessness and worthlessness.

Our first step was to find a means to ground and centre the women in order for them to regain control. We did this through breathing and physical grounding exercises, gentle hand massages (always checking out that the women felt safe with touch). Each woman had a book and in this we wrote about or drew a picture of the safe place they could find for themselves inside. For some this meant visualising a calm, secure place, for others remembering a good powerful time in their lives or finding a body position that made them feel strong. Securing these safe places was essential and gave them something to refer to outside of the group. Where necessary and possible we also arranged for them to have extra support outside. We used painting, drama and movement to enable them to express and validate the range of feelings they had in a contained way. It was very important to allow them the space to let out these feelings and not simply cover them up with reassuring platitudes. The women needed to act out or draw anger as well as sadness and fear. This both gave it an outlet and gave us a way to work with what was going on for them.

I cannot overstate the need to keep repeating the four endorsements mentioned above and to reassure the women that their feelings and reactions are normal and appropriate.

Working with strengths

As time went past I learnt to fight my own way and I learn how to become mature, to speak what I need to speak out.

Moving on from the holding phase our next task was to help the women find some order for the chaos they had felt. We acknowledged that each woman had skills and strengths. The act of surviving through the experience of sexual abuse and continuing with their lives was a certain indicator of this. So also was the living with all the societal oppressions put on them in having a learning disability. We spent a lot of time encouraging the women to recognise these strengths and get in touch with the power they have. To do this we took a step back and put the women in the context of their whole selves and their lives. Elfrida re-emerged as a sexual abuse survivor and we started by identifying her strengths and power. We then did the same for each woman, using drawings of themselves, pie charts and life maps. Collectively we acknowledged each woman's strengths and helped them recognise times in their lives when they had felt them.

It is extremely important when working with sexual abuse to put the experience into the context of women's whole lives, to help them recapture their sense of control and the dreams and aspirations they have, to reassure them that women can and do survive the experience and go on to have happy and fulfilling lives. Also that women do gain strength from surviving sexual abuse, which can never be taken away. Reading them stories written by and about survivors endorsed this as did showing the film *The Color Purple* (Angelou 1988; Bass and Davis 1988; Walker 1991). Workers must be careful when using this film to avoid colluding with racist stereotypes of black male perpetrators. We addressed this in our group by reminding them on several occasions that all but one of the perpetrators known to the group were white, asserting that perpetrators, like survivors, come from all classes, races and culture, and reinforcing this before and after the film. If there is any danger that this message will not be heard then the film should not be used.

Dealing with feelings when they arise

For several women in the group their experiences of sexual abuse kept coming up in various and often unpredictable ways. We reassured the women by saying that it was normal and to be expected, but they needed more ways of controlling these feelings. In response we found that naming and making understandable common reactions like nightmares, flashbacks and unbidden memories helped. Identifying what was happening and knowing that these were normal occurrences following sexual abuse gave them some degree of control in itself.

We encouraged the women to share these experiences when they happened, with the group. When several of the women did bring their recurrent nightmares and flashbacks to us we endeavoured to work through them. Sometimes simply talking it through was enough, but on other occasions we used a variety of ways to contain and work through it, e.g. one woman was able to banish a particularly disturbing image from her nightmares by drawing it over and over again, then with the assistance of all the women she tore the pictures up and destroyed them.

Another way we found of gaining control over feelings is to identify where they are coming from and what they are about. It can also help to differentiate feelings which come from the heart, thoughts from the head and gut reactions. This kind of information helps both the participant and the worker understand what is happening and find appropriate ways to address it.

Working with the whole woman

> Most people get sexually abused, yeah . . . you go to the police
> . . . you sit there for hours and hours . . . then they ring up a
> friend and say 'we're not going to do nothing because the people
> have got a learning disability'.

Being able to value yourself is a fundamental right for all women and intrinsic to the healing process of those who have been sexually abused. Working towards this necessitates seeing the woman in the context of her whole life, of how she may also have been oppressed by society, because of her gender, race, culture, sexuality or disability. All oppression devalues and disempowers: sexual abuse compounds and reinforces these feelings. We worked to acknowledge and address oppression the women experienced.

We spent a lot of time exploring what having a learning disability meant to the women and looking at ways to reclaim their right to be valued. The women experienced oppression in all areas of their lives and particularly from the legal system and the police. Although two women reported being raped to the police neither of the cases proceeded any further, largely due to the fact that the women had a learning disability and their statements were not taken seriously.

We all felt angry and dismayed about this and, as workers, we wanted to avoid it enforcing their sense of worthlessness and powerlessness. We affirmed that this was a blatant misuse of justice and that we should fight to make sure they were given the same rights as any other woman. First, we invited a local policewoman into the group and the women explained to her why they were angry and upset with the police. She assured us she would take this information back to her police station. Second, we concluded that before the group ended we would find a way to use our experience and get the women's voices and opinions heard.

MAKING THE VIDEO AND CLOSURE OF THE GROUP

In the two years that the group ran we slowly worked our way through most of our initial agenda. At the outset we had put a limit of two years on the group and so we were all prepared for it to end in July 1988. About six months before the ending date we looked at various ways to pursue our documenting/campaigning intention. Through a fortunate contact we were put in touch with Kim and Claire, two women film-makers known as Twentieth Century Vixen. They were looking for a women's community group to make a video with. After meeting them they decided they would like to work with us and for all the reasons I covered in my introduction to the chapter we agreed to go ahead and made a video. Not all of the women wanted to appear in the video but they all enjoyed being a part of the process.

Kim and Claire were extremely enabling film-makers to work with, they were respectful and encouraging. Despite the room being crowded with lights and film-making equipment they were able to put us so much at ease that we virtually forgot they were there. Over two consecutive weeks they filmed four hours of group discussion. From this they edited it down to twenty minutes and *Between Ourselves* (the name was chosen by the women) was made. The women had overall editorial control of the video to ensure that they were happy with the content and were not disclosing anything they did not want made public.

The women were delighted with the outcome. On their decision the video was for women only. It was meant for other women with learning disabilities and women who worked with them.

The whole process happened very quickly and we received our first responses three months before the group closed. All of the reviews were positive and as they each came out we would take pride in reading them aloud in the group. As a result the group was also approached to address conferences for people with learning disabilities, seminars for women workers and asked to meet up with other women's groups.

We felt that the group's aim to have its voice heard and campaign on behalf of all the women with a learning disability had been satisfactorily met.

This all added up to a very positive ending – we were all sad to finish but knew it was time to move on.

CONCLUSION

Two weeks before the end of the group we spent one session reviewing whether or not the women felt that the group had met the aims they had agreed on at the beginning. Overall they felt they had achieved a lot of their expectations and more. All of the women were actively more confident. Those who had been enabled to talk about their experiences of sexual abuse either inside or with social workers outside of the group had found it beneficial. They all felt that they were able to assert themselves more and had a greater degree of choice in their lives as a result of the group. Whether or not they appeared in the video they felt proud to have made it about the group and experienced it as validating and empowering.

As a worker I felt pleased with the group process and the video. However, given the circumstances of the women's lives and the range of issues that arose I think it would be naive and unrealistic to believe that the group was enough in itself. Like the women I believe all women should have access to a women's group, not just one, but several at different stages in their lives and to address different issues. I like to view our group as just the beginning of a process that, with luck and adequate resources, the women can continue.

The women in this group and the process itself taught me a considerable amount about communication, about listening and respecting the group's pace, and about the importance of being open to hear women's experiences of sexual abuse. Both professionally and personally I value the time I spent with these women.

I will leave the final remark to one of the group members:

> Sometimes it's embarrassing to talk but we want to support other women with learning difficulties. It's important to tell other people about our lives. We do have problems as well that need special help from places for women.

NOTE

1 The issue of empowerment had serious implications for us as group leaders. We attempted to address this by consistently checking out our attitudes and challenging ourselves and each other when we felt we misused the power we had. We became increasingly aware of the issue of being two white group leaders of a racially mixed group and the obvious limitations this created. In retrospect we concluded that it is vital that the leadership reflect the racial mix of the group.

The logical and most appropriate place to take any concerns is supervision. However, at the time we had no access to either internal or external supervision (the agency has since rectified this omission). So Nikki and I looked very much to each other for guidance and support. As the group developed and the focus turned to sexual abuse we found it necessary to receive outside help. Fortunately we were able to get this from other women's organisations and in particular from some workers from the London Rape Crisis Centre.

REFERENCES

Angelou, M. (1988) *I Know Why the Caged Bird Sings*. London: Hutchinson Education.
Bass, E. and Davis, L. (1988) *The Courage to Heal*. London: Harper & Row.
Between Ourselves (1988) 15-minute video for purchase or hire, Twentieth Century Vixen, 28 Southampton Street, Brighton, East Sussex BN2 2UT.
Walker, A. (1991). *The Color Purple*. Cambridge: Cambridge University Press.

8 Working with sexually abused individuals who have a learning disability

Valerie Sinason

'SHE WON'T KNOW HER ARSE FROM HER ELBOW'

'Stupid cow wouldn't know a bloody thing about it. If she can stick buttons and rubbish down her bloody gob, she won't know her arse from her elbow anyway.' Those words were uttered by a young woman with a severe learning disability in a psychotherapy session. She was mimicking with painful accuracy the male nurse who had abused her at her long-stay hospital. Not expected to understand what was happening, she understood only too well. However, her long-term emotional problems, expressed via pica, the indiscriminate swallowing of almost any substance she could find, meant that her clear communications about abuse were totally disregarded.

Children and adults all over the world face the problem of being disbelieved if they talk about sexual abuse. Women who have been raped, old people who have been physically or sexually abused and abused children are unwelcome survivors of a largely invisible crime. Their words puncture societal fantasies about community health and as punishment their experiences are too often dismissed as fantasies. Their bodies, behaviour and emotions bear the scars of trauma and are clinical proof. However, clinical proof and legal proof can be far apart and there continues to be widespread public denial of the extent of abuse.

What happens when the victims are children or adults with a mental disability? As Brown and Craft (1989) point out:

> We need to be clear at the outset that we must not fall into the trap of seeing people with a mental handicap as a homogeneous group with special problems in this respect. The abuse they experience is part of the general phenomenon of abuse. Abuse of anyone with a mental handicap does, however, present our services with special, although not unique, difficulties.
>
> (Brown and Craft 1989: 1)

There are very few statistics available on the incidence and prevalence of disability and abuse although the amount of work being done in this field is heartening, given the newness of it. In America, the Seattle Rape Relief and Sexual Assault Centre reported 700 cases of sexual abuse involving this population between 1977 and 1983. In 1984 the Cincinnati Adolescent Clinic reported that one quarter of its female patients had been abused. Individual residential schools for deaf children have reported incidences of abuse of 50 per cent (Sullivan *et al*. 1987). Generally speaking, professionals consider that abuse in the handicapped population is higher than in the non-handicapped (Tharinger *et al*. 1990; Anderson 1982). In the last six years there has been an increase in small statistical samples which add up to a disturbingly large international picture of abuse even though the main epidemiological work remains to be done (Sinason 1992, 1993).

Children and adults with mental and physical disabilities face particular difficulties when trying to tell of abuse. They are more likely to be disbelieved or even ignored. Their communication problems are exploited by their abuser who is subtly aided by many of the unthinking networks in which they exist. Those who are mentally ill in addition face even more disbelief. Out of fear of misinterpreting a psychotic fantasy of abuse, too many psychotic patients who have been abused are condemned to meaninglessness. Edward, for example (Sinason 1990), walked around a hospital ward for years, his repeated cries of 'Edward, stupid piece of shit, get under' ignored as a meaningless signature tune by caring but emotionally negligent staff. The fact that he was recounting a piece of life-history was not realised.

Communication difficulties are ironically twofold. The worker who is skilled in sexual abuse work but not in the field of learning disabilities can feel so frightened about not understanding the words or body gestures of a handicapped child or adult that she or he loses their own intelligence and avoids the work. The worker who is skilled in learning disabilities but not in sexual abuse cannot bear to believe or trust what she or he is hearing. Sometimes this is due to not bearing to hear that a child burdened by a handicap has been further burdened by abuse. The Tavistock Clinic Child Protection Training organised by Dr Judith Trowell and Ms Beverley Loughlin has been amongst the first to try and remedy this – by including a special learning disabilities component in the training.

Where the handicap is more severe there are greater communication problems which can make many workers feel extremely deskilled. The handicapped child and adult may indeed have a major problem in communicating. This makes their chance of reporting abuse less likely (O'Day 1983). However, the cause of the communication problem may well be compounded by emotional trauma. For example, Eileen Vizard (1986) drew attention to two different childhood responses to abuse. Regardless of the existence or level of handicap some children and adults are able to communicate their abuse clearly while others are extremely difficult to understand. In my experience, chronic abuse from a main attachment figure is more likely to lead to individuals falling into the second category. In addition, like Varley (1984), I have found such children and adults to be more vulnerable to psychotic breakdown as a result of abuse than the non-handicapped population (Sinason 1992, 1993).

There are several factors that make the child or adult with mental disabilities more vulnerable. Joan, for example, is dependent on others for help with basic toileting and dressing functions. This makes it far harder to her to say 'no' to surreptitious or open exploitation of these activities because without the helper she would not survive. Educational packages that talk about private parts of the body are no use to this group when their private parts have to be touched by their caretakers. Where the written content does justice to these issues, the artwork is rarely suitable for adults and if the only adult to read the education package is the abuser the situation is not moved forward. A new series of books from St George's Hospital Medical School aims to pass on such messages by the pictures (Hollins and Sinason 1992). Quite apart from penetration of orifices, an abusive experience can regularly occur when workers are consciously or unconsciously transmitting sexual feeling whilst carrying out important acts of bodily caretaking.

The difficulty in communicating verbally makes it harder for the individual with a disability to show her plight to anyone except by body language. Excessive masturbating or eroticised inappropriate behaviour is all too often dismissed as part of the handicap rather than seen as a bodily way of possibly revealing disturbing experiences. We all have available a long checklist of behaviours and bodily communications that are possible symptoms of abuse which are too often ignored when it comes to children, young people and adults with disabilities.

Unworked-through unconscious guilt about having a handicap can exacerbate a fear of abandonment, leading to greater compliance. I have frequently found in therapy that the patient with a disability has a fantasy that his handicap is the product of bad parental sex and hence he already feels linked to a disturbed sexuality. This arrests his psychosexual development and makes him more vulnerable (Sinason 1988, 1989). Fantasies about the handicap do not exist solely in the mind of the individual. Parents, workers and wider society share primitive fantasies. The birth of a handicapped baby can have a major affect on early bonding and attachment, especially when there is lack of support for parents at this time. Blacher and Meyers (1983) show how lack of attachment can lead to physical abuse. Parental guilt over producing a handicapped child can be projected onto the child who is then seen as the source of all family disturbance and a fair candidate for emotional, physical and sexual exploitation within the home and outside of it.

In the Tavistock Clinic Mental Handicap Workshop and at St. George's we assess and treat children and adults with learning disabilities who are also emotionally disturbed. Sexual abuse has been a frequent experience in our client group. Some have been referred to us because of disturbed behaviour linked to known abuse, others have revealed it during the process of an assessment or in long-term therapy.

In this chapter I would like to look at how sexual abuse affected two individuals referred for therapy. In the first example I look at an initial assessment that proved particularly successful. It highlights some of the issues I have mentioned earlier. (I have elsewhere written of assessment and treatment that proved particularly difficult or unsuccessful (Sinason 1988, 1989).)

THE MAN WHO PROPOSED TO A CHICKEN

Mr J. Jay (not his real name) was 36 years old, had a severe learning disability, and had been referred for a therapeutic assessment. This was because of his head-banging and eye-poking. He had lived with his father until he was thirty-five, when his father died of cancer. Like many people with a learning disability, his first move to 'care' represented a double bereavement, the loss of his own home and the loss of his father. He had emotionally lost his mother earlier. She left home when he was eight, had since married and moved to a different part of the country and wished for no contact with him. This loss of a history is something painfully familiar for many adults with learning disabilities and has been described by Brendan McCormack (1991) as well as Joan Bicknell (1983) and Sheila Hollins (1985) at St George's Hospital.

In the Unit he was moved to, sensitive workers made allowances for his bereavement. However, although his head-banging and eye-poking were of the greatest concern, there was also disquiet about his sexual behaviour. He would approach male and female workers by exposing his genitals and buttocks and reaching out to touch theirs. On being rejected he would become bewildered, then desperate and then start attacking himself. He also stole women's clothes from the female residents and occasionally wore female underwear. More recently he had approached a little girl and exposed himself. This had increased fears about moving him to a community home.

When I visited the home to observe Mr Jay a painful scene greeted me. It was a sunny day and the home boasted a large well-kept garden. In addition to the flourishing vegetable and flower gardens (tended by residents with the aid of a professional gardener) there were also chickens, rabbits and a tortoise. The other residents were sitting on deckchairs chatting or sunbathing. A few walked round and round the perimeter.

Mr Jay was on his own. He was walking back from the rabbit hutch to the chicken shed to the tortoise and back again. Before each animal he knelt down, unzipped his fly, exposed his penis and asked, in a most plaintive tone, 'Will you marry me?'. He knelt quietly for a moment in case a reply came. Then he stood up, adjusted his trousers and walked to the next animal where the process repeated itself.

Without the disturbing act of exposure at the end, I was witnessing a theme of some of the most painful children's stories: not belonging; the orphan who asks each kind of animal 'Will you be my mummy?' A painful burden of history transmitted itself to me in two stages. My immediate thoughts were that Mr Jay felt so orphaned by his father's death that he did not know what species he was or belonged to or, indeed, if he represented any species. He did not know if anyone or anything would ever marry him or want to be with him. He did not know the meaning of privacy. He did not know what the human act of intercourse meant.

Painful as they were, those thoughts were soon swept away by even more painful ones. Mr Jay did know. He knew very well the meaning of his isolation, disturbance, lack of sexual privacy and exhibitionism. He was showing everybody in as blatant a way as he could that someone had treated him as the wrong species, the wrong gender.

His key worker had told Mr Jay she was concerned at the attacks he made on himself and had asked a colleague to think about this with her. She gently approached him as he adjusted his trousers and waved goodbye to the tortoise. Standing quite a long physical distance from him she told him her colleague had arrived and asked if he would like to come and talk with us. He came up to me and one hand quickly went to his fly. The worker quickly said 'No, this is a visitor', unfortunately rather implying that otherwise such behaviour was all right!

Inside a pleasant staff room we all took a seat. Mr Jay was a slender, well-dressed man with a thin, anxious face that did not keep still for a moment. His face was a mirror of both his own speedily changing inner conversations and the expressions on my face and his worker's. I was quite amazed at the accuracy of these mimicking expressions. In the midst of these a formal sentence would emerge like 'I don't mind' – like a remnant from another life or someone else's head.

I asked his worker about him and how she saw his problems while he stroked the faces of women in the magazines lying on the table. She described how his father's death had made a huge impact on him as he had lived with his father all his life. His father was the only relative he had who cared for him and now he had no visitors. While he was still at home social workers had noted that there was a problem with him stealing women's clothes but he had never exposed himself before. In addition to that, they had had to curtail his outings because if they went anywhere where there was a woman's shop he would steal soft underwear and slips. Finally, he had damaged one eye by his poking and concussed himself with his head-banging.

After 25 minutes I asked Mr Jay if he felt he would like to spend some time talking with me by himself. He nodded, but as his worker got up to leave he looked quite anxious and stood up too. She explained that I would see him just for half an hour and then she would come back again. Relieved, he sat down.

When she had gone he immediately picked up the bag of objects I had brought and carefully took everything out. There were crayons, pens, paper, plasticine, magazines, small toy animals and people and some doll's house furniture. Where there are severe communication difficulties I find it helpful to provide for adults a range of concrete objects. Mr Jay was instantly drawn to the mother doll. As his workers had said his mother had rejected him I asked what the doll was he had picked up. 'Mother', he uttered. He had quite a severe speech defect but managed to make himself clear. I agreed, noting to myself that he was aware of gender and age differences.

He felt the doll's skirt very tentatively and then more and more urgently as if he was trying to work something out from the feel of the material. I said he was in the room with a new woman, Mrs Sinason, and perhaps that made him think of his mother. He nodded and continued feeling the skirt with quite a rapt wondering expression on his face. I said he was touching the mother doll's skirt very carefully. We knew his mother had left him when he was a very little boy.

Perhaps he felt more attached to his mother by her skirt than anything else.

He listened quite sadly and then picked up a little girl doll and fingered her skirt and slip. This did not convey a sexual communication but a rather deprived one.

I said he was very interested in the feel of the material. He nodded. I said his worker had commented he mainly stole soft underwear. He agreed. I wondered if his mother had worn soft pants and slips like that. 'Yes. I don't mind.' I said he had all these phrases to say he didn't mind when he did mind and had rather sad thoughts really.

His face continued to change its expressions rapidly and then a rather perverse expression appeared while he fingered the dolls. I said first he longed for something soft and silky and mother-like but now he wanted to have those things in a different way. He picked up a baby boy doll. He looked disparagingly at the baby boy's lack of petticoat and threw him away.

I said that he had been the only child – perhaps his mum and dad had wished he was a girl. 'Yes', he said clearly, with no speech defect. He looked at me most intently. 'Did your mum ever dress you as a girl?', I asked. There was no reply but he picked up the baby boy again. He looked at me intently, leaving me in no doubt that he wished me to be his voice and continue. 'Did your dad wish you were a girl?', I asked. 'Yes', he replied, very clearly and loudly.

There was a painful pause. I said I wondered if anyone had wished he was a girl or a lady at night-time. 'Yes', he said intently, and picked up a cot to put the baby boy in. Then he looked at me most clearly and intelligently and laid the father doll on top of the baby boy. He looked at me with all mimicry of my expressions gone.

I said it looked as if there was a man who thought the baby boy was a woman at night-time. 'Yes', he said – again intensely, and wanting me to continue. 'I wonder who that man is?', I asked. 'Dad', he shouted. Then his face went into thousands of changes again, including mimicking of my expressions and banging his head. 'It's all right though, really', he repeated, his speech defect returning as he banged his head rhythmically. I said it was a terrible blow to him what had happened with his dad and just thinking about it made him wish he could bang those memories out of his head.

He stopped banging his head but looked round to the door repeatedly, waiting for his worker. I said he had done enough work and he nodded. I asked if he would like me to tell his worker what we had discussed. He nodded. It was then time for her to return.

When she came into the room he relaxed in his chair but the

intelligence had left his face and it had become a mimicking mirror again. I said there were two strands on my mind connected with Mr Jay's problems. First was how deprived he had felt of motherly attention and how touching and having soft things was a way of being with and having that mother. The key worker agreed she had seen that strand. I said second, there was the question of whether anyone wanted him as a girl or used him as a girl. Had she ever thought of sexual abuse?

She instantly said she had thought about it a lot with the father but had never mentioned it. Mr Jay looked at her quickly and then went back to copying expressions. She said an old social work report mentioned that his father used to buy him pornographic magazines and soft frilly underwear. 'I think social services ignored it because they were just glad his father looked after him. People must have thought his father was doing that to keep him happy rather than to . . . encourage it.'

I said it seemed to me that Mr Jay was indeed upset about his father's death. He had lost someone who had been his most important and consistent family member. However, he had also lost something bad as well as something good and now he was realising that things he had to do with his father were not good for him and this was very distressing. I suggested that Mr Jay was asking the chickens to marry him because he wanted everyone to see that he had been treated in a terrible way. He had had to be with his father the way only a wife should and that was as mad as a chicken and a man marrying each other. Mr Jay nodded and said, 'But it's all right though, really it is. I don't mind.'

His worker said he had had years of minding and not being able to stop anything so it was not surprising he had given up. But now he was showing he did mind. She asked him if he would like to meet me to discuss these matters each week. He nodded.

In fact he only saw me for six sessions. He wanted a chance to think about his father and how much he missed him, as well as to consider the bad things his father had done. Shengold (1979) has commented that:

> If the very person who abuses and is experienced as bad must be turned to for relief of the distress that the parent has caused, then the child must out of desperate need register the parent delusionally as good.

Mr Jay needed to come to terms with the two experiences he had of his father, the abuser and the good father. His self-injury stopped dramatically and on the sixth session he said 'Enough'.

A year later I heard that Mr Jay had returned to his challenging behaviour after his key worker left. Once the new one settled in his equilibrium returned after a few weeks of eroticised behaviour. Mr Jay is likely to remain vulnerable, especially at times of change. However, the thoughtfulness of the staff meant that his behaviour was understood to have meaning. Mr Jay did not need or want long-term therapy. He wanted his communication to be understood.

For every Mr Jay I see whose communication is clear to me there are also, of course, those whose struggles to communicate I do not understand. In my clinical notes of work I undertook before 1983 I can now vividly see the examples of abuse that I was blind to then. However, what Mr Jay highlights for me is the way in which communications are explained away because the painfulness of the abuse is not tolerable. As a therapist exploring his communication I had the freedom to be his voice and verbalise what my clinical experience taught me was his meaning. Those essential clinical questions I asked would, in a legal context, be seen as leading questions and dismissed. Whilst the particular communication needs of those with physical impairments and learning disabilities are denied in law there will be more Mr Jays, burdened by their own lifetime ghosts, unable to move on.

'IF YOU TELL, YOUR PARENTS WILL DIE'

Miss Karen Kay (not her real name), a young woman with a severe learning disability, was referred at the age of nineteen by her mother. She had been relatively content in her different school settings apart from a period of depression when her father died of a heart attack when she was ten. At eighteen she and her mother made a major decision to aid her independence. She went to live in a group home and began to attend a new Adult Training Centre whilst coming to live at home for weekends and holidays.

After a couple of months Mrs Kay noticed a dramatic change in her daughter. She lost interest in all the subjects she had previously enjoyed. She clung to her mother during her weekends home and cried desperately saying she did not want to go back. Against the advice of the social worker, who considered it important for Miss Kay to manage the first separation, Mrs Kay took her back home. However, this did nothing to alleviate her terror at going to her Adult Training Centre.

Mrs Kay received little sympathy for that predicament. The social worker, upset at her client's deterioration, told Mrs Kay that she had hindered her daughter's first independent steps in group living and now they were paying for it as Miss Kay was no happier even though she was at home. The mother then insisted that her daughter go back to the group home.

For the period of one year Miss Kay deteriorated. She either stayed quietly withdrawn in her room when visiting her mother at weekends or she would start shouting. She would kick fences, bus-stops and shop windows and her Training Centre reported that she was very difficult to manage there with explosive violent outbursts. In fact, she needed to be removed from group rooms regularly as she was so difficult to manage. Mrs Kay grew increasingly distressed but agreed with the social worker that Miss Kay would eventually have to adjust. A psychiatrist consulted by the mother prescribed tranquillisers. Nobody considered there was any meaning in Miss Kay's behaviour other than 'settling-in difficulties'.

One morning, whilst Mrs Kay was on a shopping trip with her daughter, she was shocked to hear her shout crudely to a complete stranger, 'I'll pull your knickers down, play with your fanny, see how you like it'. The language and tone were initially shocking but they illuminated the past year's behaviour in a worrying way. At home she asked her daughter why she had said that. She then heard a painful story. According to her daughter, a worker at the Training Centre, one she was most attached to, had been abusing her from the month she began. He would take her into any empty room and order her to lift up her dress and pull down her knickers. He would then touch her vagina roughly and insert his fingers. This was accompanied by ferocious talk of how bad she was. He would then tell her to turn round, anally penetrate her and finally beat her buttocks with a ruler. He told her this was because she was so bad and naughty. He told her not to make a noise but to 'take it like an adult' and gave the additional warning that her mother would die if she told her.

Mrs Kay believed her daughter completely. She could see how her distressed behaviour and emotional deterioration had led to outbursts at the Centre where the Instructor was gratefully seen as a disciplinary aid in removing her from the large group. No-one considered anything that happened unusual. Because Miss Kay's behaviour was only seen in terms of an inability to settle in, her increased emotional disturbance was ignored. Each time she was removed from the room by this worker other staff were grateful.

The moment Mrs Kay heard an articulate account from her daughter she understood the meaning of all she had witnessed over the year.

She felt devastated. Although she had worried about her daughter's state she now felt guilty for having allowed her to return again and again to the place of abuse. She called the social worker, anxious to bring the whole matter out into the open. The social worker was shocked at the suggestion and said it must be a fantasy of Miss Kay's. When a meeting was arranged with the Head of the Training Centre Miss Kay was unable to speak and the Head dismissed her story as a fantasy.

The violation of abuse applies to the network as well as the child or adult. To know that a trusted colleague has been implicated is a devastating experience for a staff group and support is needed for them too. Whether a colleague is rightly or wrongly named the work environment becomes devastated.

Mrs Kay, with the aid of her married son, withdrew her daughter from the place she no longer trusted and wrote to the local police. The police were sympathetic and made a preliminary investigation. However, one person's word against another's with no corroborative evidence could not be taken any further. It is important to note how grateful Miss Kay and her mother were for the sympathetic response of the police. There was medical proof of anal penetration but that did not show who the rapist was. Miss Kay grew more depressed, made animal noises, had violent outbursts and was unable to do anything without her mother. This was the point at which Mrs Kay referred her daughter for therapy.

The referral letter, in addition to relating the details of what had happened, added that Miss Kay was now deeply disturbed, had nightmares, was wetting and smearing and kept her light on at night.

First meeting

They arrived on time. Mrs Kay, clearly under a great deal of strain, sat protectively on one side of her daughter. She was an elegant woman in her late forties, dressed in subdued colours. Miss Kay, on the other hand, wore brighter colours appropriate to her age. She looked at me eagerly as I approached and, unlike many other adults with a handicap, she did not break into a bright, beaming false smile.

After I had introduced myself and asked how they would like to be addressed, we went to my room. Miss Kay made clear she would like her mother to speak first. The mother, in a quiet distressed way, recounted all the background details I have mentioned. Miss Kay nodded approvingly as her mother spoke and, from time to time, added her own comments. 'It is not right. My body is private. Bad.

You can't do that to me.' I said she really knew now how to protect herself. She agreed proudly.

After half an hour I suggested that Miss Kay and I spoke on our own, if she felt comfortable about that. She agreed and her mother left the room. I asked her to come back in twenty minutes.

When she had left the room Miss Kay turned urgently to me. 'Mr X did that to me on Monday, Tuesday, Wednesday, Thursday, Friday. He did it in September, October, November, December, January, February, March, not in Easter, May, June, July, not in summer.' I said she knew all the days of the week and all the months of the year accurately. She nodded. 'Yes. I know a lot and I know what Mr X did. Mr X mustn't stay in his job. He needs a smack and the sack and a thing in his bottom-hole.'

I said she really wished he could know what it was like to be her and lose what mattered. 'Yes. Because you can't pull your knickers down and lift your dress up. No. It's private. Private body.' I agreed and said she really knew now what was private.

'Bad, bad, bad Mr X', she said. She cried. 'And I am not there and he is.' I said that felt so unfair that he was still in his job and she was out of her centre. 'Yes. Bad. Bad. Never again. I'll scream next time. I'll scream. Scream. Like in the Centre.'

I said she screamed in the Centre but not when she was alone with Mr X. 'No. He said "Don't scream. Be quiet. Or it will be worse. Take it like an adult".' I said he had told her not to scream and she had screamed instead at other people. 'Yes. Why?' I asked what she thought. She screwed up her fists and shouted, 'Bad, bad, Mr X. Bad. Private. Never again. Scream.'

I said she found it very painful now realising what he had done and how she had not screamed. She wished she had screamed while he did it. 'Yes', she whispered. Then she really amazed me by saying, 'It was exciting. I thought I liked it and then I didn't and it hurt'. She looked at me intently. 'It hurt me and I didn't want to like it and I didn't because it hurt but it still excited me.'

I said that was very important; it told us one reason why she was so upset now. 'Yes. Bad Mr X. He shouldn't do things to hurt people and he shouldn't make me like it and hurt me. Bad. Private body. Not pull down your knickers. Not ladies, not men, not boys, not girls. Private. Front-hole and bottom-hole private.' I agreed and repeated that now she really did know what was private. But what Mr X had done had hurt her really badly, not just because he had hurt her private body and done things he should not, but because she felt bad she had liked it sometimes and she felt bad she had not screamed.

'Yes', she whispered. 'I screamed after and I screamed before. And once Mum knew it stopped. If she knew January it would have stopped January and if she knew February it would have stopped February. But she did not know then and I didn't know then and it went on Mondays and Tuesdays and Wednesdays and Thursdays and Fridays.' I said it really did sound as if it went on and on horribly for her in the Centre and it still was going on horribly round and round in her head.

'Round and round. Never again. My private body.'

There was a knock on the door and her mother came back in. I asked Miss Kay what she would like me to discuss. She said she wanted me to make sure the man went to prison so he could not hurt other people.

Session 2

At our second meeting Mrs Kay and Miss Kay both looked pale and exhausted. Mother said her daughter had deteriorated dramatically in the week. She was talking about what had happened all the time, over and over again.

'All the time, round and round and over and over', agreed Miss Kay. I said it was such a terrible experience to have gone through that only now were we beginning to see the full force of it. Miss Kay said she would like to see me on her own for half an hour and we agreed her mother would return then.

On her own Miss Kay said, 'I am going to self-defence, judo, karate, never again. Not touch me. No-one touches me. I am private. All of me is private. My face is private, my eyes are private, legs private. Don't touch. Keep out. Not allowed. Never again. I will shout. I will shout in the park. I will shout on a bus. I will shout on a train. All the time. He said I must not shout. Now I shout, shout, shout all the time. Even if it hurts my voice I shout. Shout, shout. Never again. Never be quiet'. I said she would really shout if it ever happened again but the trouble was she was shouting everywhere. She was so upset she had not shouted at the man she was shouting all the time to make up for it. 'I did shout', she said. Then she was quiet and wiped a tear. 'I didn't shout. "Be quiet", he said. He said be quiet and not tell mother. Never tell mother. "Never speak. Bad girl. Bad. Take it like an adult".'

Session 3

On the third session I was extremely worried for Miss Kay. Immensely hurt that nothing had happened to the man, she was in a florid psychotic state for most of the session. 'Not hurt. Bad. People in cars. Dangerous. Don't touch my hand. Dangerous body. Hands are private. Don't hurt. Not allowed. Never. Shout. All the time. Walls, doors. Don't touch. Never. Not allowed.' Her mother said she had been in this state all week at home. On the few occasions they had gone out she had shouted at anyone who came near her in the shops.

I suggested we try and video a statement about the abuse next week in the hope there would still be some clarity left and Miss Kay was extremely keen on the idea.

At the end of this meeting Miss Kay made clear she would like weekly therapy for herself and her mother said she would be able to bring her. We decided that we would video Miss Kay speaking so that was available for possible future investigation and then therapy could proceed.

Session 4: Video meeting

To my surprise Miss Kay arrived looking most purposeful and stating proudly she was going to say everything that happened. She pointed to her smart new clothes and her carefully combed hair. I said she felt better inside now we were going to make a video and that had allowed her to make her outside smarter. She agreed. 'Video and get the man a sack, a smack. Then it can go to court and I will stay in court and I will tell the judge everything, everything, everything so he doesn't do it again to other people.' I had anatomically correct dolls available to help her communicate.

VS: We are now starting from the beginning and we are talking about what happened on the video so we have it as clear as we can.

KK: He did bad things to me, like that down there. (She picks up a female doll, bends it over and hits its bottom. Then she picked up a male doll and made him put his penis in the girl doll's anus.)

VS: He has put his penis in her bottom-hole and hit her bottom.

KK: And I'm older than him.

VS: How old is he?

KK: I don't know. I am only nineteen at the ATC.

VS: You were nineteen when you went to the ATC and now you are older so you feel older than the man.

KK: Yes, and if he tried it again I'd go to my mother. He said you don't tell your mother – that is what he said but I do, I go and I went to my mum. I can't go to my dad because he is dead. But I tell my brother, my mother, straightaway and I went to you and I told you and I told the policeman straightaway. I wasn't making any noise. No noise. Nothing.

VS: Maybe you wished it was straightaway but it wasn't straightaway.

KK: I was a lot frightened I was . . . .

VS: You didn't tell your mother straightaway but you did tell her after, and your brother.

KK: Yes. I did tell them after. He said don't tell but I did. I told my mum and my brother.

VS: What did you tell them the man had done? Will you say it again for the video?

KK: He done bad things to me and hurt me.

VS: He did.

KK: Yes he did. He hurt me so much. (She bends the doll over and points to its bottom.) He put me like that and did it – bang and he put his penis in and hurt me and that did hurt – and he hit me again and he said 'Don't tell your mum'.

VS: It is hard, like the smile now, because you felt a bit excited as well as frightened.

KK: Yes.

VS: And that made it worse after.

KK: Yes. And nothing happened because he said he didn't. He hurt me on my front side too. Inside. Where the wee comes. He made it go funny and then he said I was bad. 'Don't tell your mother and father. They'll die.' I said my father was dead. He said that was because I was bad and if I told my mother would die too because I was bad and that was why he did it.

VS: You were frightened you were bad for getting excited and because your father was dead.

The video session lasted an hour and in it Miss Kay managed to tell me more of the time of day it happened, the room it happened in and what her abuser looked like when he was excited. Although I held in mind the possibility that Miss Kay might be linking her abuse to the wrong person, I did not doubt the authenticity of her story. In thirteen years of working with abused children and adults I have yet to come across a false reporting of rape or abuse. Only on two occasions has there been a cause for concern. In both those cases the children (one handicapped and one not) transferred the real abuse onto a less frightening figure with the same emotional authenticity. They were too terrified of the real abuser to name him. I have always kept open that small possibility of naming the wrong person since then. To be wrongly accused of abuse can sometimes be almost as traumatic as being abused.

After the video session Miss Kay experienced a week of relief. She managed to express herself clearly. Then a period of grief began. Her mother reported she had stopped making animal noises. However, a week of crying began.

Session 5

Miss Kay wore a low-cut dress and gazed at her breasts on the way up the stairs. 'I look pretty', she announced. Inside the room I suggested she was concerned I would not care about what was inside her, only what she looked like on the outside. 'Pretty', she repeated looking down. 'Hurt me', she said, putting her hand on her bottom. 'Bad. Go away. Private body.' I commented she was showing me and herself another private part of her body – her breasts. She was looking to make sure they were all right and did not hurt. Perhaps she worried they were not pretty as the man had not been interested in them. 'No. He didn't look', she said sadly.

I suggested she was missing the man because even though he hurt her and excited her in a difficult way he also looked at her private body. 'Yes. And he mustn't look. Why didn't he look at them?', she asked plaintively, gazing down at her breasts.

A meeting with her mother after the next session revealed that Miss Kay was masturbating publicly, in shops and parks, wherever they went. For the next few months therapy centred on Miss Kay's perpetuation of abuse via her own handling of herself.

Session 20

Miss Kay sidled onto her seat in an extremely sexual way. She placed a hand between her legs and looked at me with an excited smile. I commented on this. She looked sad and removed her hand. Then her hand travelled like a magnet towards her bottom. She touched her bottom and grinned excitedly and then looked upset again. I said she was really struggling between a Miss Kay who had got excited by the man and a Miss Kay who hated having got excited. 'Yes. Bad. He should be in prison for that – making me like it.' I agreed with her that one of the worst aspects of the abuse was that she had developed a taste she would not have had. 'No. Grown ups don't do that, not to themselves, not to children. Not right. Private. He did it. He told me not to tell. He said my father died because of me. He said don't tell. You're bad. And he excited my front and back.'

Session 30

By Session 30 a new Centre had at last been found. However, instead of feeling relieved Mrs Kay was terrified. 'My daughter was trusting and sexually innocent when she started that Centre. Now she knows too much and the worst thing is she misses it and the man, and when she goes to a new Centre she will find someone to do it to her – whether it's a teacher or a student.' Like her daughter, she sadly added, 'You know, that is the worst thing he has done, making her have to like it'.

For a few weeks Mrs Kay kept her daughter at home to protect her but she realised that added to Miss Kay's depression. Finally she let her go. Her concerns were only too fully realised.

Session 35

Miss Kay came in with a low-cut blouse and tight trousers. She giggled when she saw me and sidled on to the chair. 'Masturbating isn't private', she said, 'so long as it is friends and not the man it is all right.'

I said she was telling me masturbating was different when she wanted it to happen but asked why she did not think it was private?

'Because I can do it with my friends in the coffee breaks and lunchbreaks at my new Centre. It is nice. Everyone does it. They can look. It is not private. The man isn't here. The teachers don't do it so it is all right.'

For a moment I was paralysed. In my mind I was weighing up issues to do with the rights of people with handicaps to a sexual life and accommodation to abuse, exploitation. Finally, I commented, 'It was so horrible that the man did it to you without you choosing, you want to do it yourself whenever you can with friends you choose'. 'Yes', she agreed, 'because it is not private because everyone does it at my new Centre.'

Session 40

As we got to grips with Miss Kay's damaging attempt to wipe out the abuse by replicating it under conditions of her own choosing, she became both more depressed and violent. Her mother found it impossible to take her out to visit relatives and friends as she started shouting at them again.

In Session 40 she came in dressed in a very dowdy way and began a litany – 'I want it to happen to my mother. I want the man to do it to her. I want him to do it to my uncle. I want him to do it to my nieces and nephews. They should all be locked up in prison and arrested. My mother should be arrested because she is like the man and so are you and so are all the teachers at the new Centre. I want to be the man and have a penis and do it to everyone on their fronts and their bottoms with no clothes on. I will tell them all not to tell and I will tell them all their father will die'.

The next term consisted of working on her guilt about her father's death and her hurt at having a handicap. Her eroticised behaviour began to diminish. After a year and a half the flavour of the session was very different:

Session 50

She came in wearing a dress I had not seen before and sat down on the armchair facing me. (Not surprisingly she has not wanted to lie down on the couch.) 'My dad died when I was ten. I am twenty.' I agreed and said she was now twice as old as she had been when he died. 'Yes. I am older now. I am older than the man too.' I said she was much older than when she had been abused by the man and perhaps she wished she was older than him too. 'Yes. Because if I was older than him he couldn't do it to me. He only did it because I was younger. . . .' There was a painful pause. 'And because I'm handicapped.'

I asked why she thought that. 'Because I didn't know I could tell because he said I shouldn't tell. I would have told if I didn't have a handicap.' I said that may have made it harder for her to tell but people without handicaps also found it hard to tell when they had been abused. She looked interested in that but then pursued another train of thought.

'If I wasn't born like this my father wouldn't die.' I said she seemed to think her handicap had made her father die. She nodded vigorously. Then she burst into tears. 'My mother said it. She said it.' I asked what her mother had said. 'She said – "Shut up! Stop making a noise, you bad girl! You will give your father his death! It's bad enough without that noise".' She sobbed bitterly.

I thought with her about how those words had stuck in her head and prevented her screaming when the man hurt her. She also made clear that she understood the sophisticated communication in, 'It's bad enough without that noise'.

Only after we had looked at the guilt she carried for her handicap and her father's death could we properly tackle how the abuse had built its home on that fertile soil.

CONCLUSION

Miss Kay will remain vulnerable despite her hard work in once-weekly psychoanalytic psychotherapy. Mr Jay will also remain vulnerable. Both suffered the tragedy of having their disability exploited. Although both were verbal they had severe learning disabilities and were thereby less at risk than those with multiple and profound disabilities. Nevertheless, the repercussions of their experience of abuse were enormous. Mr Jay and Miss Kay, against their wish and will, had been made addicts. They had been injected with perverse and sadistic experiences that they could only find relief from in disturbed eroticised behaviour. Unlike those with profound handicaps they at least had verbal language to help them communicate. In the BAPSCAN Working Party on Disability and Abuse convened by Margaret Kennedy of Keep Deaf Children Safe, we have been hearing the even more painful stories of children and adults whose life-stories can only be conveyed by their body movements. Nevertheless, the increasing awareness of the impact of abuse on individuals with mild and severe learning disabilities will surely help to highlight the vulnerability to exploitation of all those who need the security of safe others to live their lives. The launch of NAPSAC and VOICE sine this chapter was first drafted herald a hopeful new era.

REFERENCES

Anderson, C. (1982) *Teaching People with Mental Retardation about Sexual Abuse Prevention*. Santa Cruz: CA Network Publications.

Bicknell, J. (1983) 'The psychopathology of handicap'. *British Journal of Medical Psychology* 56, 167–8.

Blacher, J. and Meyers, C. (1983) 'A review of attachment formation and disorder of handicapped children'. *American Journal of Mental Deficiency* 87 (4): 359–71.

Brown, H. and Craft, A. (eds) (1989) *Thinking the Unthinkable: Papers on Sexual Abuse and People with Learning Difficulties*. London: Family Planning Association.

Cincinnati Adolescent Clinic (1984), quoted by Kennedy, M. (1990) in *Keep Deaf Children Safe* (KDCS), Nuffield Hearing and Speech Centre, Grays Inn Road, London.

Hollins, S. (1985) *The Last Taboo*, video available from Mrs Freda Macey, Dept of Mental Health Sciences, St George's Hospital Medical School, Cranmer Terrace, London SW17 0RE.

Hollins, S. and Sinason, V. (1992) *Jenny Speaks Out* and *Bob Tells All*, St George's Hospital Medical School: Sovereign Series.

McCormack, B. (1991) 'Thinking, Discourse and the Denial of History: Psychodynamic aspects of mental handicap'. *Irish Journal of Psychological Medicine*, 8, 59–64.

O'Day, B. (1983) *Preventing Sexual Abuse of Persons with Disabilities: a Curriculum for the Hearing Impaired, Physically Disabled, Blind and Mentally Retarded Students*. Santa Cruz: CA Network Publications.

Seattle Rape Relief Centre (1983), quoted by Kennedy, M. (1990) in *Keep Deaf Children Safe* (KDCS), Nuffield Hearing and Speech Clinic, Grays Inn Road, London.

Shengold, L. (1979) 'Child abuse and deprivation: soul murder'. *Journal of the American Psychoanalytical Association* 27: 533–99.

Sinason, V. (1986) 'Secondary mental handicap and its relationship to trauma'. *Psychoanalytic Psychotherapy* 2 (2): 131–54.

Sinason, V. (1988) 'Richard III, Echo and Hephaestus: sexuality and mental/ multiple handicap'. *Journal of Child Psychotherapy* 14 (2): 93–105.

Sinason, V. (1989) 'Uncovering and responding to sexual abuse in handicapped patients in psychotherapeutic settings', in Brown, H. and Craft, A. (eds) *Thinking the Unthinkable: Papers on Sexual Abuse and People with Learning Difficulties*. London: Family Planning Association.

Sinason, V. (1990) 'Individual psychoanalytical psychotherapy with severely and profoundly handicapped patients', in Dosen, A., Van Gennep, A. and Zwanniken, G.J. (eds) *Treatment of Mental Illness and Behavioural Disorder in the Mentally Retarded*. The Netherlands: Logon.

Sinason, V. (1992) *Mental Handicap and the Human Condition: New Approaches from the Tavistock*. London: Free Association.

Sinason, V. (1993) 'Abuse and disability', in Hobbs, C. and Wynne, J. (eds) *Child Abuse. Ballière's Clinical Paediatrics*. London: Ballière Tindall.

Sullivan, P.M., Vernon, M. and Scanlan, J.M. (1987) 'Sexual abuse of deaf youth'. *American Annals of the Deaf* 132 (4): 256–62.

Tharinger, D., Horton, C.B. and Millea, S. (1990) 'Sexual abuse and exploitation of children and adults with mental retardation and other handicaps'. *Child Abuse and Neglect*, 14: 301–12.

Varley, C.K. (1984) 'Schizophreniform psychoses in mentally retarded girls following sexual assault'. *American Journal of Psychiatry* 24: 293–311.

Vizard, E. (1986) 'Interviewing young sexually abused children'. *Family Law*, 313: 28–33.

ADDRESSES

NAPSAC (National Association for the Protection from Sexual Abuse of Adults and Children with Learning Disabilities)
Dept. of Learning Disabilities
Queens Medical Centre
Nottingham NG7 2UH

VOICE
P.O. Box 238
Derby DE1 9JN

9 A model clinic approach for the reproductive health care of persons with developmental disabilities

Thomas Elkins

INTRODUCTION

An interdisciplinary model clinic for the consideration of reproductive health, sexuality and socialisation concerns has been established now for several years at both the University of Tennessee and the University of Michigan in the United States. These were established in response to the unique set of reproductive health concerns that the population of those with mental handicap/developmental disabilities presents to the obstetrician/gynecologist. Such concerns were once considered to be limited to mental institutions. However, in a time of non- and de-institutionalisation, increased socialisation, increased community involvement and improved educational and medical prognosis, the health care problems of the adolescent and adult with mental disabilities will probably be encountered with increasing frequency by the community-based physician. The two model clinics were, therefore, established in an effort to provide a standard of care which could be replicated and taught to physicians attempting to provide care for these patients in community as well as university-based programmes.

Before the establishment of either clinic, discussions were held with parent support groups, health care providers and educational professionals concerning the best method to organise such a health care delivery system. Other similar clinic efforts had met with little success in the past because of a strong focus on family planning which emphasised the very controversial areas of sexuality, contraception and sterilisation (David *et al.* 1976). A more global clinic system that would offer gynaecological care in general, as well as a focus on socialisation and sexuality, was developed.

FORMATION OF AN ETHICS COMMITTEE

Before patients were ever seen, an advisory or ethics committee was formed at each clinic location (Elkins *et al.* 1986a, 1986b). This committee consisted of leadership from within the community who had a known interest in persons with developmental disabilities. Committee members included attorneys, clergy, social workers, group home supervisors, professional educators, special education experts, parents, members of advocacy groups and developmentally disabled persons themselves. These groups decided upon a set of principles for patient management that were based upon ethical concerns. These included:

— The basic commitment of the clinic was to provide care that is in the best interest of the patient.
— Each patient was to be treated as an unique individual with distinct problems regardless of their level of mental retardation.
— Each problem discussed was to be viewed as only a portion of the patient's total reproductive health concerns being addressed by the clinic (for example, hysterectomy might solve the problem of menstrual hygiene but would do nothing to combat recurrent sexual abuse and alone would not be a comprehensive approach to sexuality and reproductive health concerns for many patients).
— Each therapeutic intervention should provide the least restrictive means or least harmful alternative form of care whenever reasonable.
— Decisions should be made in a manner sensitive to widely shared societal views and to the fact that these views are pluralistic (for example, therapeutic decisions whenever possible should be opened to the review of an ethics/advisory committee composed of societal representatives who have an interest and expertise in mental retardation).
— Certain procedures or therapies, such as surgical sterilisation, require review by a committee because of the problem of informed consent in this population (Elkins *et al.* 1986a).

THE WORK OF THE CLINIC

With these guidelines, a clinic was established within the Department of Obstetrics and Gynecology. The following data concern the clinic established at the University of Michigan which began in 1985. Within six months after the establishment of such a clinic programme, the clinic was filled to capacity on all clinic days, and it has remained full for at least six to nine months in advance since that time. A regular gynaecological clinic for persons with developmental disabilities occurs each Thursday from 5 to 7.30 p.m. During that time, approximately six to ten patients are seen by a staff that includes a nurse specialist, a social worker, a nurse's aide, a clerk, a staff physician in obstetrics and gynaecology and a resident physician from the same department. One Thursday evening clinic out of each month is set aside as a sedation clinic in which patients who are impossible to examine without sedation receive pelvic examinations without excessive force or coercion. The entire clinic programme includes daily counselling sessions that are provided by the social work staff connected to the clinic. Group counselling programmes are held on Friday afternoons in conjunction with local group homes and school facilities. Once a month, on Wednesday evening, the advisory committee for the clinic meets to discuss particular aspects of patient management and to review requests for invasive surgical procedures such as sterilisation.

Over 500 patients have now been seen in the overall clinic programme. Although the brevity of this chapter does not allow a full discussion of all aspects of the clinic programme, highlights of patient presentations and clinic management will be presented in the following discussion.

Numerous groups of patients have been identified by the reason for their visit to the clinic. The need to have routine care provided has been the most frequent reason for a visit to the clinic. In most states in America, a full physical examination, including a pelvic examination, is mandated by state law for adult patients. Most gynaecologists begin seeing patients for examinations in the United States when they become sexually active, when they begin experiencing regular menses or difficulty with menses, or when they reach adulthood and receive examinations as part of premarital evaluations, school or employment evaluations or insurance evaluations. It was notable that in the population of persons with developmental disabilities, pelvic examinations were often never done. If they were performed, they were often done in clinics where large groups of patients were examined in a harsh, very physical and very rapid fashion. In a review of the first 167 women appearing in the clinic, approximately 100 of these patients had never had a pelvic examination. Eighty-seven of the patients had severe or profound handicaps and had been seen by physicians on multiple occasions but had always had the pelvic examination deferred (Elkins *et al.* 1988b).

The overall programme to accomplish pelvic examinations in

difficult-to-manage patients with mental retardation involves several aspects. Pre-examination counselling by the clinic nurse and social worker is done to assess barriers to the pelvic examination that would include fears, anxieties and past experiences on the part of the patient that might make an examination difficult. Many times, physical problems and deformities make pelvic examinations awkward and a great deal of care must be taken in positioning the patient to accomplish a pelvic examination without harm. A socialisation/sexuality assessment is also provided for those patients who have the mental capacity to respond to a pictorial questionnaire about the appropriateness of social behavioural patterns. This has been helpful in planning a total care programme for the patient and in identifying patients in whom sexual abuse has already occurred.

The pelvic examination itself may have to be modified in order to be accomplished in many patients. Only 26 (17 per cent) of the first 167 patients allowed a complete pelvic examination including speculum insertion, but 91 (58 per cent) allowed a bimanual examination with a Q-tip swab of the cervix placed in the cervical os by digital direction (Elkins, McNeeley *et al.* 1988b). Twenty-five of the first 167 patients required sedation with either Ketamine or Midazolam. Since this initial report, over 100 patients have received sedation for pelvic examinations with an 85 per cent success rate in providing safe and diagnostically accurate pelvic examinations in an outpatient setting. Pelvic examinations have been diagnostic in this population, revealing five patients with greatly enlarged uteri due to leiomyomata, and three patients with large ovarian neoplasms.

Discussions are currently under way about the necessity for pap smears on an annual basis in this population group. At the present time, data are being collected to justify the more liberal use of pelvic ultrasound for follow-up visits on an annual basis after an initial complete pelvic evaluation (including a pap smear) has been accomplished. This greatly simplifies the examination process and does not appear at this time to subject patients to unnecessarily high rates of diagnostic inaccuracy. The current clinic protocol calls for a full examination on initial presentation to the clinic, followed by bimanual or ultrasonographic evaluations for at least two to four years before another full examination is done including another pap smear, when patients are not sexually active. Certainly sexual activity, a history of precancerous conditions of the cervix, excessive vaginal bleeding or discharge or suspicion of pelvic malignancy would call for annual or even more frequent complete pelvic examinations with pap smears and other diagnostic procedures, as indicated.

One of the largest groups of patients in the clinic programme is those who have presented with the complaint of premenstrual syndrome ('PMS'). Premenstrual syndrome has become a very popular condition in the United States and 53 of the first 350 patients coming to the clinic presented with 'PMS' (Elkins 1988). The symptomatology in these patients is somewhat unusual in its severity. Sixteen showed very aggressive, self-abusive behaviour. Fifteen presented with severe agitation on several days prior to each menses. Twelve had extreme crying and mood changes. Five showed excessive anxiety around menses and eight had an increase in seizures during menses. Two actually had excessive vomiting around all of their menstrual cycles. Forty-eight of these patients were either severely, profoundly or moderately mentally handicapped. A request was made for care-providers to bring a menstrual and behavioural calendar to the clinic on each clinic visit. In keeping with the above management principles for the clinic, initial therapeutic approaches were aimed at treating milder symptomatology with Vitamin B6 supplements, mild diuretics and dietary/exercise changes. These measures were almost universally ineffective in those with severe and profound handicaps. Non-steroidal anti-inflammatory agents were used to eliminate any suspected dysmenorrhoea and this was thought to be helpful in a few patients. It was usually necessary to try to modify or eliminate cyclic hormones to achieve any markedly noticeable therapeutic success in this patient group. This was accomplished with low-dose oral contraceptives, continuous oral progestin therapy or, on occasion, the use of Depo Provera intramuscularly. At the current time, this remains one of the more difficult areas to manage and other ways are being sought to control the PMS-like symptoms in this population group.

Extreme cramping and noticeable pain with menses without other associated symptoms were found in only 8 of the first 350 patients. These were almost always treated successfully with non-steroidal anti-inflammatory agents or low-dose oral contraceptives.

However, patients with irregular menses made up 49 of the first 300 plus patients studied. Again, 36 of these 49 had severe or profound mental handicap. Surgical correction of this problem was not the first step in management of irregular menses. This is, at least in part, because of the high number of associated medical problems that are usually found in this population group, which makes surgery a higher risk (McNeeley and Elkins 1989). Seizure disorders were noted in 22 of these patients, five were hepatitis B carriers, six were quadriplegic, five had severe scoliosis, five had Down's syndrome and numerous other medical problems were noted in the remainder of the patients. Management of patients who presented with almost daily irregular vaginal bleeding included the use of progestin-dominant low-dose oral contraceptive pills, continuous oral progestins or, on occasion, even Depo Provera. This, when coupled with menstrual hygiene training for both the patient and their care-providers, gave excellent results in almost every instance.

Sixteen patients presented with severe hypermenorrhoea (excessive bleeding with periods). Six of these patients had moderate mental handicaps while seven had either severe or profound mental handicaps. In these patients, menstrual hygiene was often a severe problem for care-providers or families. In more than one patient, extreme hygiene problems were complicated by the presence of a hepatitis B carrier state, making menses a definite health hazard for those attempting to provide care and supervision for the patient. Hypermenorrhoea is also more difficult to manage medically. Despite attempts to control heavy menses with low-dose oral contraceptives, menstrual hygiene training, continuous progestin therapy, or even surgical dilatation and curettage, hysterectomies were performed in eight patients. Five of these patients had leiomyomata uteri with greatly enlarged symptomatic fibroids, and three had refractory heavy menstrual bleeding that responded well to vaginal hysterectomy.

The use of Depo Provera has been controversial in persons with mental retardation. It has been brought before the advisory/ethics committee for discussion in both of these clinic settings on numerous occasions. A review of the first twenty-four patients receiving Depo Provera showed that ten of the patients were being tried on Depo Provera for severe, refractory PMS-like symptoms including increased seizures with menses and severe self-abusive behaviour. Refractory menstrual hygiene problems were reasons for resorting to Depo Provera in six patients and refractory bleeding was the reason for resorting to Depo Provera in eight others. The medication appears generally to be very well tolerated with minimal side effects (Chamberlain *et al.* 1984). However, numerous patients develop almost daily spotting and bleeding for the first months on Depo Provera and its usefulness will be questioned in the future as newer medications become available to manage irregular bleeding problems and cyclic behavioural problems in persons with intellectual disabilities. Only two patients developed any degree of lethargy or depression that was noticeable on Depo Provera. Hot flushes occurred in one patient. However, seventeen of the first twenty-four patients complained of irregular and occasionally heavy breakthrough bleeding. Lipid profiles are being checked routinely because of the theoretical risk of hypercholesterolemia and hyperlipidemia developing in patients who are given long-term continuous progestin therapy. However, the physicians working in the clinic programme have consistently suggested that trials of Depo Provera are more reasonable than resorting to hysterectomy too quickly in patients with vaginal bleeding problems. Out of the first thirty-five patients who received major surgery within this clinic population, aspiration pneumonia (in four patients), post-operative faecal impaction, pelvic cellulitis, urinary tract infection and small bowel obstruction were all identified as post-operative complications (McNeeley and Elkins 1989). Therefore, surgical therapy is considered a method of treatment of last resort for patients with gynaecological concerns.

Requests for sterilisation were also seen in twenty-three of the first three hundred patients. Interestingly, eighteen of these twenty-three patients had mild or moderate mental handicaps and eighteen lived with their family while two others lived in foster care with other families. This is in marked contrast to the remainder of clinic population sub-groups in which patients with severe and profound retardation abound and in which most patients are noted to be living in group home facilities. All requests for sterilisation are submitted to the advisory/ethics committee and to the legal counsel of the hospital prior to proceeding. Requirements for sterilisation in the model clinic at the University of Michigan include:

1) That the patient be 'of legal age' to normally be considered for such a decision.
2) That the patient was, had been or anticipated being sexually active.
3) That the patient be permanently mentally handicapped.
4) That the patient be physically capable of pregnancy.
5) That other methods of contraception had either been tried or were considered medically unreasonable in a particular setting.
6) That the patient exhibits some evidence of positive decisional-capacity including the ability to determine that they did not want to be pregnant, that they did not want children and that they did understand that a surgical procedure would be necessary to achieve their request for sterilisation.
7) That the patient had not been adjudicated mentally incompetent and that no legal guardian was trying to provide secondary informed consent on behalf of the patient in the sterilisation request.

These requirements are in agreement with Michigan State Law that disallows operations for sterilisation alone upon guardianship approval when a person is mentally incompetent (Elkins, Hoyle *et al.* 1988a).

SEXUALITY COUNSELLING PROGRAMME

Perhaps one of the more interesting parts of the entire clinic programme has been the socialisation and sexuality counselling component directed by Sally Kope, MSW. Out of the first 400 patients, 103 persons were referred for socialisation or sexuality counselling (Edwards 1979, 1988; Edwards and Elkins 1989). Thirty-eight of these were referred for basic socialisation and sexuality education including thirty-two from group home programmes within the area. The majority of these were managed in group counselling sessions utilising a multitude of teaching materials that included a strong reliance on audio-visual works. Twenty-nine of the patients were referred for social/sexual behavioural problems including nineteen who had been involved in inappropriate touching in local school, sheltered workshop or group home facilities. Four were accused of sexual abuse and two had been identified for going with strangers or for indulging in excessive amounts of public masturbation. Self-exposure and obscene phone calls were also noted in this initial sub-group of twenty-nine individuals. All of them required prolonged individual counselling that emphasised repetitive educational messages and behavioural modification techniques with the co-operation of the community. All have been markedly successful to this point. Reproductive health issues, including questions about marriage or pregnancy, occurred in only thirteen of the referrals. Problems with family stress were noted on only five occasions and these were managed by family interactional counselling sessions.

A recounting of some presenting situations underscores the need for such counselling services. One 35-year-old woman with Down's syndrome was capable of working in a professional's office, typing fifty words per minute and exhibiting excellent verbal expression. However, she had no socialisation or sexuality training and was frightened by the aggressive behaviour of male friends with whom she partially undressed to watch television videos. Another 18-year-old young man was accused of abusive behaviour because he persisted in publicly kissing a high-school cheerleader despite requests to leave her alone. The counselling task became twofold: to assist him in re-directing his socialisation efforts and to help him through the grief response encountered when he realised the reality of his handicap and of the fact that many 'normal' acquaintances did not consider him a desirable peer. Another 21-year-old man first requested a sex change operation. On further counselling, it was apparent that he was being chided by peers because of gynaecomastia caused by long-term Dilantin therapy for seizures. Simple mastectomies were success-fully suggested with counselling to clarify the young man's requests and reassure him of his worth. Other cases, reported in other publications, only further emphasise the need for social-sexual coun-selling services as an essential feature of a reproductive health programme for persons with developmental disabilities. Issues such as abortion, sterilisation, family stress, homosexuality, sexual abuse, etc. became steady concerns in such a programme.

The most striking sub-group within the socialisation and sexuality counselling programme were those individuals who had been sexually abused. Thirty-three of the first one hundred and three patients referred for counselling had been sexually abused in the past. Seven had been victims of rape, ten of incest and sixteen of other forms of sexual abuse. Great efforts were made not only to assist them in identifying abusive behaviour, but in teaching sexual abuse avoidance practices such as the knowledge of private versus public behaviour, body parts, times, places and language. Efforts were made to reinforce avoidance of strangers in public places, 'buddy' behaviour in public, appropriate greeting behaviour and displays of affection. Sexual abuse remains a significant problem for persons with developmental disabili-ties and much greater efforts will be required in the future to improve in this area of care for such individuals.

CONCLUSION

The model clinic programme described here has provided the founda-tion for the teaching of not only gynaecological care, but biomedical ethics, and socialisation and sexuality for persons with developmental disabilities and for the 'normal' population as well. The clinic at the University of Michigan continues to expand with the potential for routine dental examinations becoming a possibility in the near future on sedation evenings when patients who are generally unexaminable are receiving routine health care. Many questions still remain. The advisory/ethics committee is assisting with a long-term project to define more clearly the decision-capacity necessary for informed consent in persons with mental retardation. The appropriate use of the pap smear, pelvic ultrasonography and sedation in performing routine gynaecological exams still needs clarification. Issues surrounding a growing geriatric population of individuals such as those described here will become more prominent in the future. Other issues such as sterilisation and the appropriate use of such medications as Depo Provera and such surgical procedures as hysterectomy have been and will remain controversial within this population group. However, efforts continue to evaluate and re-evaluate the clinic programme so that optimum care can be provided in the most humane and compassionate fashion.

REFERENCES

Chamberlain, A., Rauh, J., Passer, A., McGrath, M. and Burket, R. (1984) 'Issues in fertility control for mentally retarded female adolescents: sexual activity, sexual abuse, and contraception'. *Pediatrics* 73: 445–50.

David, H.P., Smith, J.D. and Friedman, E. (1976) 'Family planning services for persons handicapped by mental retardation'. *American Journal of Public Health* 66 (11): 1053–7.

Edwards, J.P. (1979) *Being Me: A social-sexual training guidebook*. Portland, Oreg.: Ednick Communications.

Edwards, J.P. (1988) 'Sexuality, marriage, and parenting for persons with Down syndrome', in Pueschel, S. (ed.) *The Young Person with Down Syndrome*. Baltimore: Paul H Brookes.

Edwards, J. and Elkins, T.E. (1989) *Just Between Us: A guide to the socialisation and sexuality training of persons with mental retardation (for parents and professionals)*. Portland, Oreg.: Ednick Communications.

Elkins, T.E. (1988) 'Premenstrual syndrome: a problem occasionally for persons with Down syndrome, too'. *Down Syndrome News*: 19–20.

Elkins, T.E., Gafford, L.S., Wilks, C.S., Muram, D. and Golden, G. (1986a) 'A model clinic for reproductive health concerns of the mentally handicapped'. *Obstetrics and Gynecology* 68 (2): 185–8.

Elkins, T.E., Strong, C., Wolfe, A.R. and Brown, D. (1986b) 'An ethics committee in a reproductive health clinic for mentally handicapped persons'. *Hastings Center Report* 20–2.

Elkins, T.E., Hoyle, D., Darnton, T., McNeeley, S.G. and Heaton, C.S. (1988a) 'The use of a societally based ethics/advisory committee to aid in decisions to sterilise mentally handicapped patients'. *Adolescent and Pediatric Gynecology* 1: 190–4.

Elkins, T.E., McNeeley, S.G., Rosen, D., Heaton, C., Sorg, C., DeLancy, J.O.L. and Kope, S. (1988b) 'A clinical observation of a program to accomplish pelvic exams in difficult-to-manage patients with mental retardation'. *Adolescent and Pediatric Gynecology* 1: 195–8.

McNeeley, S.G. and Elkins, T.E. (1989) 'Gynecologic surgery and surgical morbidity in mentally handicapped women'. *Obstetrics and Gynecology* 74: 155–8.

10 HIV/AIDS and safer sex work with people with learning disabilities

Michelle McCarthy and David Thompson

THE AIDS AWARENESS/SEX EDUCATION PROJECT

This chapter reports on the work of the authors through the AIDS Awareness/Sex Education Project, which carries out safer sex work with people with learning disabilities. It describes some of the major issues that arise out of that work.

The AIDS Awareness/Sex Education Project was set up in 1989 from funds made available by the Department of Health for HIV prevention work. The project's brief was to develop sex education and HIV work with the residents of three large hospitals for people with learning disabilities, with a population of 1,600, in Hertfordshire (now the Horizon NHS Trust).

The project has also worked to a lesser extent with staff and people with learning disabilities in community settings and this chapter is based on that combined experience.

The team has three full-time staff and its work can be divided into the following areas:

Individual work

This entails working on a one-to-one basis with people with learning disabilities. It is important to state that this work is dominated by referrals concerning sexual abuse: both of women and men who have experienced, or who continue to experience, abuse and of men with learning disabilities who sexually abuse others. Individual work takes the pattern of weekly sessions over the medium term, that is from two to eight months.

Group work

This involves running women's and men's groups to discuss and give information about different aspects of relationships and sex. The groups run for approximately ten to twelve weeks.

Staff training

The aim of this is to develop staff's awareness of the issues and to develop their confidence to undertake sex education work.

Policy development

Guidelines and policies are produced for staff in the three hospitals.

Consultancy

The project offers consultancy on matters relating to HIV and sexuality of people with learning disabilities on a local, regional and national basis.

The key features of the project's approach to sex education are:

— a commitment to equal opportunities. In practice this means that providing both partners are consenting the project team does not value any one kind of sexual relationship above any other
— working from a feminist perspective. In practice this means acknowledging the usual inequality of power between women and men in sexual relationships. (For further discussion see McCarthy and Thompson 1991.)

The authors have developed educational and training materials based on these principles (McCarthy and Thompson 1993).

HIV AND SAFER SEX EDUCATION

Recognising that people with learning disabilities have sexual experiences with other people means recognising that there is a risk of HIV infection. Research in the United States (Kastner *et al.* 1992) and anecdotal evidence in this country shows that although the numbers are small, some people with learning disabilities have been infected with HIV. Although the sexual behaviour of most people with learning disabilities does not put them at particularly high risk, there is still justification for targeting them with special safer sex educational initiatives. This justification comes from the generally poor access people with learning disabilities have to general HIV information (perhaps through limited reading skills and/or through limited understanding of things they may have heard on television).

Responsible safer sex education should not be done in isolation, but should ensure that people with learning disabilities have general information and skills regarding sex and sexuality. Also such education should be sensitive to the actual pattern of HIV infection and therefore regard as a priority work with men with learning disabilities who have sex with other men.

One of the first steps in safer sex work is to decide what information or advice people with learning disabilities should be given. Over the years many safer sex messages have been given to the public. Some of these messages comment on what relationships people should be in to have sex, for example, 'wait until marriage', 'stick to one partner' or 'cut down on the number of partners'. Some safer sex messages suggest who sexual partners should and should not be, e.g. to 'know' your partner and to avoid having relationships with bisexual men or prostitutes. Some safer sex messages relate to specific sexual acts, e.g. 'use a condom', 'avoid anal sex', 'oral sex is risky'. (NB These examples are to illustrate the complexity of safer sex information and are not necessarily ones with which the authors agree.)

When working with a person with learning disabilities it is obviously necessary to decide which of the many messages are to be given. The reasons for this are twofold: first, to sort those which give useful information about HIV transmission from those which have more to do with morality, and second, because people with learning disabilities may not be able to make sense of what could be conflicting and unclear information. What this means in practice is that the safer sex advice given could be different or at least modified for individuals with learning disabilities, depending on their levels of ability and understanding.

It can be difficult for some workers to see their role as one that filters information to people with learning disabilities instead of aiming to provide them with as much information as possible. However, prioritising and simplifying HIV information and safer sex messages has proved to be very important with most people with learning disabilities. In general safer sex education, a lot of attention is given to establishing the difference between HIV and AIDS, and language which compounds these two is rejected (e.g. 'AIDS virus'). However, our experience is that very few people with learning disabilities have been able to understand the difference between HIV and AIDS, and more importantly, few would benefit greatly from understanding the distinction. Although AIDS is not an inevitable consequence of HIV infection and many HIV health educators would reject presenting the message that 'AIDS equals death', we agree with Jacobs *et al.* (1989) that sometimes accuracy may have to be sacrificed for the sake of getting the message across. What is necessary is that a person with learning disabilities has a clear idea of the potential outcome of unsafe sex. Many of the people with whom the project has worked already know that people could get AIDS from sex and people with AIDS die, which is a very useful summary.

After deciding what information to give a person with learning disabilities about safer sex, the worker needs to be aware of how much that information is stressed. Does the worker say, for example, 'If you have sex, you could use a condom' or 'You must use a condom or you'll get AIDS and die'?

The weight given to safer sex messages will be determined by how the worker sees their role. The spectrum of positions ranges from one which only wishes to give information, leaving the choice whether to have safer sex with the person with learning disabilities, through advising or encouraging/discouraging certain behaviours, to telling the person what to do. HIV counsellors and workers with people with learning disabilities may share a reluctance to direct people's behaviour or influence their choices.

However, if a 'non-directive' position is chosen, the following needs to be acknowledged: first, that this is a very difficult position to take because just raising the issue of the risk of HIV with a person with learning disabilities is bound to weight the 'choice' in favour of safer sex. Second, and more importantly, this position means leaving total responsibility for the risk of HIV transmission with individuals who may be in a very poor position to take such responsibility.

We have seen our role as advising and directing people with learning disabilities regarding safer sexual behaviour and have done so in the belief that service providers have some responsibilities in this area when people are unable to make difficult and complex decisions for themselves. This will be clarified later in the chapter.

RESOURCES

There are now a number of specialist resources available to assist in this work; namely videos, educational packages and leaflets. Most simplify information by referring to AIDS and not HIV. All of them either advise or insist on condom use (the only choice for the person with learning disabilities is to ignore that advice), e.g. one video states 'If you do choose to have sex you must use a condom' (Young Adult Institute 1987).

The resources differ greatly in what kinds of sexual activity are discussed or portrayed. Some resources only portray sexual relationships between women and men (e.g. Islington Working Group 1990). Others cover same sex relationships in a minimal way, for example one line drawing of an androgynous looking couple hugging, which effectively allows same sex relationships to be ignored (BIMH Working Party 1989). Others openly acknowledge and show intimate contact in same sex relationships (Young Adult Institute 1987; FPA of New South Wales 1990).

The sexual activities which are excluded in some of these resources reflect more upon the producers' own values and attitudes to sex. Those which do not deal with same sex relationships, or acknowledge that men have anal sex with women, do not reflect the reality of the sexual lives of many people with learning disabilities and so are unlikely to be very effective teaching aids.

It is not surprising that the HIV resources present such a restricted view of sexuality when the few resources available to date for general sex education with people with learning disabilities have traditionally only portrayed penetrative vaginal sex.

In all the resources the strongest safer sex message is to use a condom, regardless of the sexual relationship the person with a learning disability is in. We take a similar position because it does seem appropriate to encourage condom use, irrespective of the nature of the relationship, because of the potential benefits in reducing the risk of HIV and other sexually transmitted diseases. However, some people are encouraged more strongly to do so than others because of the perceived risk of HIV infection.

Advising the use of a condom for oral sex is argued for by those packs which acknowledge its existence. This is partly because of the real (though small) risk of HIV infection from oral sex, and because it may simplify the safer sex message, i.e. whatever kind of sex, always use a condom. To expect people with learning disabilities to make sense of the actual risk of oral sex does seem unreasonable when very well-informed health educators are split over how serious the risks are. This leaves the options of advising condom use or disregarding the risks. We have adhered to the latter of these strategies, telling people with learning disabilities that oral sex on a man is something which does not require a condom. The defence for this is that:

— the risk of HIV infection from oral sex is very small compared to the risks from anal or vaginal sex and priority should be given to those sexual acts with the greatest risks

— condom use for oral sex has not been taken up by the general population and it is not reasonable to have higher expectations of people with learning disabilities than of anyone else

— it allows for unprotected oral sex to be suggested as a safer sexual practice for those times when a condom is not available.

We see our responsibility as recommending the most practical strategy for HIV prevention based on the knowledge of how sex actually happens rather than on strategies which theoretically remove all risk of HIV infection.

PRACTICAL ISSUES

Three examples of the project's safer sex work with people with learning disabilities are described below. It will be seen that the work is intimate and explicit and starts with an exploration of what kind of sex the person is having and how that happens. This is done to inform the strategy for HIV prevention and to avoid making assumptions about whether the person does or does not enjoy the sex and whether they have any control over what happens.

Example 1

John is a man with learning disabilities in his thirties and he was referred for sex education after he had been picked up by police for hanging around a public toilet that was known to be used by men to meet men for sex. It was believed John had had some sexual contact there and a year ago he was picked up by the police for the same thing. At that time the response was for staff at his hostel to tell him not to go to the toilets. However, John continued to spend a lot of time out of the hostel by himself.

   Communication with John was difficult and discussing sex with him was made much easier by using line drawings of different sexual acts between men. It took eight sessions to build up the following picture of John's sexual activity. John would go regularly to the toilets where he waited until a man approached him for sex. John never exercised any choice over who his partner was. Largely, the sex involved John having the other man's penis in his mouth and/or John would masturbate the other man. On the occasions when anal sex took place it was always John who was penetrated. By establishing who did what to whom, it was possible to see that John was either giving or receiving whatever sexual acts were demanded by the other men and that John was not making any choices of his own. The pattern of behaviour did not in any way reflect John's preferences for certain sexual acts. Rather it was a powerful indication that he was being exploited. (NB This pattern has been seen in *all* the men with learning disabilities who met men for sex in public toilets or similar settings with whom the project has worked.)

The work on safer sex started by checking to see if John already knew what a condom was. He identified it as something that one man had used when he had anally penetrated him, but worryingly this was the exception. John had no idea of how to put a condom on a model penis and he had not heard of AIDS.

John was taught that if a condom was not used he could get AIDS and die. He was taught that a condom should be used for anal sex and which man has to wear it. He practised putting a condom on the model but it was apparent that he lacked the fine motor skills to do this satisfactorily.

Work was focused on negotiating safer sex, that is, teaching John what he should do if the other man was going to penetrate him without a condom. For example, because John's communication was so limited he was taught a set phrase to say to the other man: 'must use a condom or get AIDS', and John was also taught that if condoms were not available, oral sex or masturbation were safer alternatives. After approximately eight months John had learned to make the right responses to questions but it was increasingly apparent that he had very little understanding of the risks he faced and how very unlikely it was for him to be able to negotiate safer sex.

An indication of his lack of assertiveness skills was when he was asked what he would do if anal sex was hurting him (this was likely owing to his partner's insensitivity and the absence of lubrication). John's response, which probably reflected his experience, was to do nothing, accept the pain and wait until the man had finished.

Alongside the HIV work attention was given to other sexually transmitted diseases. John was taken for a checkup at a special clinic and a hepatitis B vaccination was arranged.

The conclusion of the work was that precisely because of his degree of learning disability, John was in no position to negotiate safer sex and so responsibility lay with the service providers for preventing the risk of HIV infection and for protection from sexual exploitation. However, little action was taken by the services, partly because of disbelief about the sexual behaviour and also an inability to discuss such difficult sexual behaviour.

Example 2

Tina, a woman with learning disabilities in her late twenties, was referred for sex education by the staff of the hostel where she had lived for eighteen months. Since she had arrived from a long-stay hospital, staff knew she had had a number of boyfriends. Her hospital notes described her as being 'promiscuous'. Tina had been on the pill for many years, so staff were not concerned about pregnancy, but they were worried about her risk of HIV infection. They felt that because she obviously enjoyed a lot of sex, she should be educated about the health risk and learn how to use condoms.

During the course of sex education sessions, Tina was encouraged to talk about the kind of sexual activities which took place and also to talk about who her sexual partners were. Mostly, her sexual partners were men with learning disabilities, whom she met at the hostel, day centre, social club, etc., but some were men who did not have learning disabilities, e.g. whom she had met at a holiday camp in the summer. The sexual activities were usually penetrative, both vaginal and anal. Tina said that she did not like anal sex, because it hurt, but she let the men do it. The only thing she would not let them do was put their penis in her mouth, because she believed 'it's disgusting'.

By helping Tina to talk about the details of her sexual life, it was possible to build up a good picture of what actually happened, which is essential when trying to do safer sex work. It emerged that Tina had very little control over what happened to her sexually – the men decided what kind of sex took place and Tina tolerated sex which she did not enjoy. The focus of the sex education sessions shifted from the narrow concern on referral regarding risk of HIV, to helping increase Tina's self-esteem and assertiveness skills. It was recognised that Tina would never be in a position to negotiate, much less insist on, safer sex with men until she understood that her role in sex was not simply to service men's sexual desires. As Tina had in the past refused oral sex, this was used as a good example of her asserting herself and used to try to help her build on this success in other areas.

After weekly sessions lasting some 4–5 months, Tina had learned about the need to use condoms and could put them on a model. She knew, in theory, that she did not have to have any kind of sex that she did not want. In practice, however, she was afraid to challenge the men in any way, in case they became verbally or physically abusive and/or left her. The sex education sessions ended with the concern that Tina would not be practising safer sex and would remain vulnerable to exploitation.

Example 3

Bob, a man with learning disabilities in his thirties, lived in a hostel and had a girlfriend with learning disabilities who lived in a nearby group home. They met at college and were very attracted and attached to one another. Bob was referred for sex education because he had told his key worker that he was having sex with his girlfriend. Bob had had a few girlfriends before and when he lived in a previous hostel had been known to have sex with other male residents.

In the sex education sessions Bob said that he had had vaginal intercourse with his girlfriend only a few times. He was reluctant to say where this took place because he thought staff would not like it. They were afraid of being interrupted and 'caught' by staff. Other times they kissed and touched intimately. Bob said that his girlfriend liked having sex. This was followed up by asking how he knew she liked it. He could not answer this, so was encouraged to think about what she might or might not like, and to ask her what she liked. He was told that the vagina could get sore during sex and how this could be prevented.

Bob had heard of AIDS, but did not know much about it. He learned about the need for condoms and how to use one. He became very competent at putting a condom on a model penis. He was encouraged to practise using condoms when masturbating and from his reports about this there was confidence that he was actually able to put them on himself (which could have proved to be more difficult than on a model). Because buying condoms would have taken up a significant proportion of Bob's weekly income, the hostel staff got free supplies from their local Family Planning Clinic.

The sex education worker arranged with Bob's key worker that he would provide ongoing support – reminding Bob on a regular basis that condoms should be used and being available for any problems that might arise. The sex education sessions ended with a recognition that Bob was in a good position to take on the responsibility for having safer sex. The sex education worker then did some work with the hostel staff to help them recognise *their* responsibilities – namely that Bob was much more likely to be able to put his new knowledge into practice if he and his girlfriend had some private and dignified space for sex and were not forced to snatch opportunities where they could.

SUMMARY OF BARRIERS TO A SUCCESSFUL OUTCOME

The examples above illustrate some of the reasons that attempts at teaching safer sex may not be wholly or even partially successful. These reasons have more to do with the circumstances in which people with learning disabilities live rather than the skill of the teacher. It is important to be sensitive to these so that efforts can be made to overcome them.

In our experience, the main barriers are:

— the low self-esteem of many people with learning disabilities. In order to be motivated to protect your own health (and that of your peers) there must be a belief that you are a person worth looking after and a person who *could* achieve this.
— the general lack of sex education offered to people with learning disabilities. This means that many such individuals, both women and men, do not realise that sex is meant to be a pleasurable and safe activity for both partners. It also means that some sexually active people with learning disabilities do not realise that sex can have potential consequences.
— people with learning disabilities often have to face a lack of support from staff and other carers in matters relating to sexuality. Consequently, many people with learning disabilities have developed a very strong sense that sex is not something to be discussed.
— many people with learning disabilities, whether in hospital or community settings, do not have any private places in which to conduct their sexual lives. Being forced to snatch opportunities as they arise does not give ideal circumstances for practising safer sex.
— many people with learning disabilities lack power in relation to their sexual partner, because of their gender and/or level of ability. It takes two to practise safer sex and many people (with or without learning disabilities) find it difficult or impossible to negotiate this.
— the fact that people *do* have learning disabilities and very often significant communication difficulties makes the work harder than it would be with many others in the general population.

RESPONSIBILITY AND RISK ASSESSMENT

In two of the three case studies above, it is clear that even after considerable input, the person with learning disabilities is not left in a position where they can take full responsibility for protecting their own health. In the third example, even though Bob was capable and motivated to take responsibility, he was constrained by the limitations placed on him by service providers.

We suggest that one traditional model of safer sex education with the general population, that is giving people factual information and then leaving them to 'sink or swim' with it, is not a responsible course of action when it comes to many people with learning disabilities. The obstacles or barriers to safer sex mentioned above *must* be recognised and acted upon, not glossed over. It does no service to people with learning disabilities to naively assume that by showing them a video or leaflet and teaching them how to use a condom, they can and will practise safer sex from then on. Simply giving people information about HIV/ AIDS and some practical skills is *not* enough to achieve lasting behaviour change, whether they have learning disabilities or not.

When it comes to people with learning disabilities, staff have a duty to promote and protect their clients' health and wellbeing. Under the principles of normalisation, it has long been recognised that some calculated risk-taking is appropriate in many areas of people's lives. This is also the case when it comes to sexual activity and its associated risks. However, if the conclusion at the end of some sex education work is that the individual with learning disabilities is not in a good position to take full, or even partial, responsibility for safer sex, then some assessment of risk is needed to determine if any, or what, further action is necessary.

To assess a person's risk of HIV infection, the following factors need to be examined:

— the kind of sexual activity taking place
— the person(s) with whom the individual with learning disabilities is having sex
— the frequency of the sexual contact.

The combination of these factors may indicate that, were the sexual activity to continue, there would be a very significant risk of HIV infection (if indeed the person is not already infected). Alternatively, it may be indicated that although the person is sexually active, their risk of HIV infection is very low. It is important to gauge the actual risk of HIV infection for an individual beyond simply identifying that a person has unprotected sex. This approach reflects the pressure by groups such as the Terrence Higgins Trust's Gay Men's Health Education Group for general HIV prevention work to recognise that some people, i.e. men who have sex with men, are more at risk than others.

When making their assessment of risk, staff should consider the following points:

— almost all sexual infections are caused by unprotected penetrative sex, vaginal or anal, and the receptive partner is at greater risk. Staff should not automatically assume that all sexual contact involves penetration. However, in our experience, sex involving women with learning disabilities is almost always penetrative (always vaginal and very often anal) and that when men with learning disabilities are having sex with men more able than themselves, the sex is very often penetrative and it is almost always the less able man who is penetrated.

— people with learning disabilities are unlikely to be at risk of HIV infection if they have only had sex with known people who themselves are unlikely to have HIV. For example a woman with learning disabilities having sex with her first boyfriend, who has only had one or two other women with learning disabilities as his previous sexual partners, is at very little risk.

— unusual or isolated incidents which are unlikely to re-occur should not give rise to over-reaction. For example, if a woman with learning disabilities, who normally receives high levels of super-vision, is raped by a stranger, then this should not cause very great worry in terms of risk of HIV infection, although obviously the abuse itself is of enormous concern.

— the assessment should be sensitive to the local pattern of HIV infection. This means acknowledging that in Britain men with learning disabilities having unprotected sex with unknown men who do not have learning disabilities will arouse the greatest concern, particularly in areas of high HIV incidence.

If the risk assessment process concludes that a person with learning difficulties is at low risk of contracting HIV infection, then there seems no choice for staff or carers other than to accept the situation and perhaps offer more, ongoing sex education. It may also be possible and appropriate to initiate work with the individual's sexual partner(s).

If the risk assessment process concludes that a person with learning disabilities *is* at significant risk of HIV infection (or may already be infected), then clearly some difficult decisions have to be made. It is not a responsible course of action to do nothing except worry and hope that everything will be all right.

There are two options and ideally both should be explored, as they certainly are not mutually exclusive. The first is to renew all efforts with safer sex education with a view to reducing the risk of the sexual activity. Extra resources and specialist advice will probably be necessary. If this is not successful and it seems unlikely or impossible to reduce the risk of the sex, then the second course of action may be required – this aims to help the person with learning disabilities avoid the high-risk situations. Consideration needs to be given to finding ways of stopping the person having sex which puts them (or others, if they are already infected) at risk of HIV. This is a very difficult decision to take and involves balancing an individual's right to sexual expression with the service's responsibility to protect them from unacceptable dangers. Steps aimed at preventing a person from having sex may include providing them with stimulating alternatives at times when high-risk sex would normally occur, increasing supervision levels, finding alternative residential/day placements, even using legislation to restrict a person's movements. Whilst some of these are drastic and seem undesirable actions to take, it must be remembered that HIV infection is a very serious concern. It involves a potentially life-threatening disease and these actions are only suggested for consideration when a person with learning disabilities demonstrates that they have little or no understanding or control over whether or not they might acquire it.

On one or two occasions we have identified that the risks of HIV were significant enough that action needed to be taken to prevent a man with learning disabilities from continuing with dangerous sexual activity. (NB There have been no women with learning disabilities who have caused such grave concern.) In fact, services have not taken the action necessary to prevent the risks. This seems largely due to an inability to confront the reality of the sexual lives of their clients.

HIV TESTING AND INFORMED CONSENT

If a person with learning disabilities is thought to have been at significant risk of HIV infection, then sooner or later the issue of an HIV test may arise. If the person has received sex education which has alerted them to the risks, it is quite reasonable that they may want to know themselves whether they have been infected. Alternatively, carers or staff may think that the person should have an HIV test.

Under British law, nobody should be tested for HIV without their knowledge and *informed* consent (except for anonymous screening programmes). Exceptions to this unfortunately occur, but a person can sue for assault if an HIV test is performed on them without their consent.

Some people with learning disabilities clearly can give informed consent and if this is so, their consent should obviously be sought like anybody else's. And, like anybody else, they can also withhold consent. However, a problem arises when a person with learning disabilities is *not* able to give informed consent. Strictly speaking, in law it is not possible for anyone to give consent on another adult's behalf, although this often happens on a day-to-day basis. In other medical matters, doctors and health care staff traditionally act in what would generally be considered to be in the person's best interests.

Opinion within the HIV/AIDS field is divided as to the advantages and disadvantages of HIV testing and in Britain it is a decision that is largely left up to the individual concerned. Within the field of learning disabilities there is also a range of opinion about testing. For example, the Royal College of Nursing Society of Mental Handicap Nursing is adamant that only those people with learning disabilities who can give fully informed consent may be tested (RCN 1991).

We advocate a different approach and recognise that a situation may exist where a person with learning disabilities has been at significant risk of HIV infection, but they cannot give informed consent to a test. In the belief that early medical intervention and health care monitoring could be beneficial to that person if they were HIV positive, we suggest that in some circumstances it is responsible to test a person in the absence of their informed consent. The Horizon NHS Trust, in which the project is based, devised a policy to allow for limited testing of individuals who cannot give informed consent. The procedure involves going to the High Court to seek a declaration that it would not be unlawful to test. The policy is designed to safeguard the rights of the individual and to prevent the routine testing of vulnerable people. We fully support the existence of such policies, as the alternative is tests being carried out on an *ad hoc* basis, at the request of individuals who may be ill-informed or by special clinics, which, in the absence of clear guidelines, may or may not take someone else's consent.

Because of the ethical dilemmas involved when a person with learning disabilities cannot give informed consent, there is an understandable, but regrettable, tendency to overestimate their ability to consent. It is clearly a difficult task to judge whether someone can give informed consent to a complex matter like an HIV test.

As a result of our work in this area, we suggest that to be able to give informed consent to an HIV test, a person should be able to demonstrate the following:

— that the decision to take a test is a considered one, one they have thought about for a while. This is to guard against a rash decision that may later be regretted.

— that they should be able to think of (or at least understand when presented with) some reasons that the test might *not* be a good idea. If a person is unable to understand any disadvantages of being tested, it is unlikely that their consent is fully informed.

— that they should have some sense of privacy and confidentiality surrounding the test and an HIV positive status. If a person with learning disabilities tells people indiscriminately that they 'have AIDS' this is not likely to be in their best interests.

— that they have some sense of long timescales. A person needs to understand that they are consenting to a test to detect an infection which, if they have it, may not trouble them physically for many years. It is important that the person does not think that the test will tell them that they have got AIDS and will be dead in a few days/weeks.

WAYS FORWARD

If people with learning disabilities are to be helped to protect themselves from HIV infection, then it is essential that staff and other carers have an accurate understanding of how they actually experience their sexual lives. All too often an assumption is made that in the absence of any complaint to the contrary, the sex between people with learning disabilities is unproblematic. In our experience this is rarely the case, with men with learning disabilities controlling and enjoying sexual activity at the expense of their women partners. It may be stating the obvious but adults with learning disabilities are, in fact, women and men. Any sex education which does not acknowledge that as women and men they may have different needs, interests and experiences is not likely to be very useful.

It is also essential to have a greater understanding of the sexual lives of men with learning disabilities who have sex with other men. These men have as much right as anyone else to get support and respect. Instead they often face misunderstanding and prejudice which is reflected in most specialist HIV and learning difficulties resources. Staff and carers also need to be aware of men with learning disabilities who have sex with men in public toilets (known as 'cottaging'). The numbers of men with learning disabilities who do this are far greater than most would suspect and it is high-risk behaviour in many senses – in terms of HIV infection, sexual abuse and exploitation from more able men, physical violence, arrest by the police.

Staff training and support are very important in this area of work, which arouses strong emotions and anxieties. Without adequate training and back-up resources, staff quickly feel deskilled and start looking around for an outside 'expert' to come and take over. Such 'experts' are unfortunately few and far between and the reality in most places is that if HIV education is going to take place, then it will have to be done by existing staff teams, with support on HIV/AIDS matters from local health promotion departments.

REFERENCES

BIMH Working Party (1989) *Aids and People with Learning Difficulties* (series of three booklets), Kidderminster: BIMH.

FPA of New South Wales (1990) *So You Won't Get AIDS* (teaching package), Sydney, NSW: Family Planning Association of New South Wales.

Islington Working Group on HIV and People with Learning Difficulties (1990) *Learning about Condoms*. Health Promotion Dept, Royal Northern Hospital, Holloway Road, London N7 6LD.

Jacobs, R., Samovitz, P., Levy, J. and Levy, P.H. (1989) 'Developing an AIDS prevention education programme for persons with developmental disabilities'. *Mental Retardation* 27 (4): 233–7.

Kastner, T.A., Nathanson, R.S. and Marchetti, A.G. (1992) 'Epidemiology of HIV infection in adults with developmental disabilities', in Crocker, A.C., Cohen, H.J. and Kastner, T.A. (eds) *HIV Infection and Developmental Disabilities*. Baltimore: Paul H. Brookes.

McCarthy, M. and Thompson, D. (1991) 'The politics of sex education'. *Community Care* 21 November.

McCarthy, M. and Thompson, D. (1993) *Sex and the 3 R's. Rights, Responsibilities and Risks: A Sex Education Package for Working with People with Learning Difficulties*, Hove: Pavilion Publishing.

RCN (Royal College of Nursing) (1991) *AIDS – A Proactive Approach to Mental Handicap*. London: RCN Society of Mental Handicap Nursing.

Young Adult Institute (1987) *Teaching People with Disabilities to Better Protect Themselves*, video, New York: Young Adult Institute.

11 Rationale, approaches, results and resource implications of programmes to enhance parenting skills of people with learning disabilities

Alexander Tymchuk and Linda Andron

INTRODUCTION

While parenting is recognised as a right of all citizens, parenting by people with learning disabilities has and continues to be controversial (see Hayman 1990; Tymchuk *et al.* 1987). Some of this controversy has carried over from the past, but much of the information on which historical pejorative attitudes were based is replete with problems. In order to ensure that the right to be a parent is not wrongly limited for any person including people with learning disabilities, it is important to recognise the limitations of what we currently know about parenting by people with intellectual disabilities. The problems of this earlier information included limited empiricism, changes in and misuse of diagnostic criteria for mental handicap including the limited or even non-applicability of IQ to parenting adequacy/ inadequacy, lack of operationalised definitions of what constituted adequate parenting, a limited view of parenting outcome variables, lack of any systematic study of or services for parents with learning disabilities and lack of professional training related to parenting by such individuals (Tymchuk 1990a). Current information continues to suffer from many of these previous factors with a continued noticeable lack of any systematic effort for needs assessment with adequate responses to those needs. With this lack, there continues to be limited attention paid to traditional empirical principles such as operationalisation of concepts, reliability, validity and replicability of findings (e.g. Accardo and Whitman 1990; Whitman and Accardo 1990). There also continues to be the study of mothers with mental handicap only and not of the fathers of the children or current partners of the mothers; the study of only mothers who have come to the attention of agencies, and not those who do not come to the attention of agencies; and the study of mothers who have very young children and not of those with older children. Such inadequate empiricism and the unrepresentative nature of the populations studied severely limit any generalisations about the parenting of people with learning disabilities.

SENTIMENTS EXPRESSED ABOUT PARENTS WITH LEARNING DISABILITIES

Despite these limitations, earlier sentiments about such parents included that their children will be born with a mental handicap; they will have more children than other parents; those children not born with a mental handicap will be at high risk for cognitive developmental delay and for physical and health impairment; they will abuse their children; they will purposefully neglect their children; all will provide inadequate child care; their interactions with their children are punitive, non-reinforcing, restrictive and non-stimulating; and that they are unable to learn, apply and maintain adequate parenting knowledge and skills (e.g. Bowden *et al*. 1971; Brantlinger 1988; Crain and Miller 1978; Fantuzzo *et al*. 1986; Hayman 1990; Seagull and Scheurer 1986; Schilling *et al*. 1982).

WHAT WE KNOW

In spite of these earlier sentiments, we now know that the chances of parents with mental handicap having a child born with a biological condition that is associated with what society defines as mental handicap are virtually the same as those of any other parent; without supportive interventions, the children of such parents are in fact at the same high risk for cognitive delay as are the children of many people living in poverty; with adequate supports, the risk for the children of either population is significantly lessened; without supportive interventions, the children of both groups are at risk for physical and health impairment as well as emotional and behavioural delay or impairment, but with supports, these risks are significantly less; parents with mental handicap appear to have fewer children and they tend to have them later in life than do others within the general population; they are less likely to abuse their children than was once thought and where abuse does occur, it is usually as a result of another person in the life of the mother (Tymchuk and Andron 1990); they are less likely to purposefully neglect their children than once was thought but neglect does occur, largely associated with a lack of training and support (Lynch and Bakley 1989); many parents, with supports, provide adequate child care; without supportive interventions, interactions are not necessarily punitive, but are non-reinforcing, restrictive and non-stimulating, but with supports, changes can be made (Feldman *et al.* 1986; Tymchuk and Andron 1992); these changes, however, can be short-lived if there is not continuation of training; many parents with learning disabilities are able to learn, to apply and to maintain adequate parenting knowledge and skills when interventions are matched to parental learning characteristics including the use of illustrated materials, when staff are well trained and when interventions are initially intensive and then periodic for a long term. Without these latter characteristics in the interventions, acquisition and maintenance of parenting skills is limited (e.g. Espe-Sherwindt and Kerlin 1990; Lynch and Bakley 1989; Tymchuk and Andron 1988).

AREAS IN WHICH INTERVENTIONS HAVE OCCURRED

Because of the inapplicability of traditional assessment and intervention methods with, and the unavailability of assessment and interventions specifically designed for, parents with special learning needs, including those with mental handicap, a great deal of effort is needed to operationalise and validate both assessment and intervention technology for use with this population. Such empiricism is just beginning but is of critical importance in order to ensure that any failures in parenting are not erroneously attributed to the person with learning disabilities. Assessment and intervention methodologies have been developed and implemented with some success in more global efforts designed to improve behaviour of mothers with low IQs to their young child through traditional early intervention strategies (e.g. Garber 1988; Ramey and Campbell 1984; Slater 1986). Other efforts have focused upon a two-tiered system of intervention including the successful development and implementation of both assessments and interventions for adequate child health care as well as for cognitive stimulation for the children regardless of their age. This approach also provides a focus upon the environment in which the mother lives, her needs and ways in which she copes, learns and makes decisions (Tymchuk submitted a; Tymchuk 1985; Tymchuk *et al.* 1988; Tymchuk *et al.* 1990a). In this two-tiered system child safety and adequacy of health care is of primary importance and has included home danger recognition and safety precaution implementation by and with mothers with mental handicap (Tymchuk submitted b; Tymchuk *et al.* 1990b), responding to common emergencies (Tymchuk 1990c; Tymchuk 1991;

Tymchuk *et al*; 1989, Tymchuk *et al*. 1990c), child illness symptom recognition, understanding and treatment (Tymchuk submitted b), use of common home health diagnostics, use of both prescription and over-the-counter medications (Tymchuk 1990b) and use of high-risk household products (Tymchuk *et al*. 1990d).

In the second tier several studies have demonstrated that parents with mental handicap often live in unstimulating environments (Feldman *et al*. 1986 and have few supports (Lynch and Bakley, 1989), but that there can be successful acquisition of more positive behaviours toward the child by the mother (e.g. Feldman *et al*. 1986; Peterson *et al*. 1983; Tymchuk and Andron 1992), dealing with child problematic behaviour (Tymchuk and Andron 1988) and in understanding child development (Tymchuk *et al*. 1990e).

In all of these studies, however, not all parents do well enough to maintain *sole* responsibility for their children (e.g. Espe-Sherwindt and Kerlin 1990; Lynch and Bakley 1989; Peterson *et al*. 1983; Tymchuk and Andron 1990;). Alternative models in which responsibility for some aspects of childcare is assumed by a supportive other person appears to be a very viable alternative to child removal. Given the lack of attention by society to children who are removed from any family unit, maintenance within a family group whose members genuinely love the child, however limited are other characteristics of the family, still may be preferable.

CHARACTERISTICS OF PARENTS WHO DO WELL OR NOT

We also have been able to determine those parents with learning disabilities who do relatively well and those who do poorly according to some societal standard of parenting (Tymchuk 1992). These characteristics are similar, if not identical, to those of other poor parents who do or do not do well according to this standard. And, in fact, most of these factors are associated with difficulties in parenting by most people in society. Yet these questions often are solely raised within the context of parenting by a person with learning disabilities.

The characteristics of mothers with mental handicap *who do well* include such *maternal* traits as having adequate reading recognition and comprehension abilities in order to make use of traditional societal information sources including such things as parenting manuals, labels of prescription or over-the-counter medication, instructions on high-risk household products and completing complex application forms; an IQ above 60; no concomitant emotional disturbance; no concomitant medical disorder; low stress; adequate self-concept and adequate motivation. Good outcome is also associated with such *external/environmental* traits as there only being one child in the home; having a younger child; having a child without a medical or other problem; having a spouse/partner without an emotional disorder, criminal behaviour or behaviour problem including spousal abuse; having sufficient supports (social, health, financial, vocational, psychological, legal); not having been institutionalised; having had own appropriate role-models during own upbringing; having adequately trained professionals; availability and appropriateness of materials used in training; continuity of agency involvement; and having a single agency providing multiple services and/or co-ordination (Tymchuk 1990a).

Those mothers *who do poorly* are those with such *maternal* characteristics as literally no or very rudimentary reading recognition and comprehension, so that they are unable to read and understand written materials including the use of home health diagnostics such as a thermometer, prescription medication instructions, over-the-counter medication instructions, high-risk household product instructions; having an emotional disturbance such as depression or alcoholism for which attention is needed before there can be parenting skill development (Tymchuk submitted b); a concomitant medical disorder such as cerebral palsy, epilepsy, visual or auditory impairment or illness with which the mother must cope while still providing care (Lynch and Bakley 1989; Tymchuk and Andron 1988); an IQ below 60; and having high stress, poor self-esteem and low motivation, all of which may be associated with previous experiences (including incest, abuse, poor parenting models), but which impede present child care and learning. Mothers who do poorly are also those with such *external* traits as having a child with a medical or other disorder which increases the complexity of child-rearing and taxes even the most capable parent; having more than one child or having an older child; having a spouse or partner who has an emotional problem or is abusive; having been institutionalised; having been raised in a familial situation in which abuse including incest was present; not having had any parenting instruction while in public education; not having had self health care education while in public education; and not having current available familial and other appropriate, accessible and ongoing supports (Tymchuk and Feldman 1991).

SOCIETY'S RESPONSES

While there have been individual efforts across the US, in Canada and in the UK to respond to the perceived needs of this population, such efforts have been severely hampered by the general lack of interest in this population as well as active resistance to addressing the issues by those both within and without the mental handicap field. One of the major impediments may be the fact that their own parents may be unwilling to garner support for their parenting. Such lack of political activism of parents of the parents with learning disabilities regarding the needs of this group is the antithesis of how other programmes for the child with mental handicap, autism or other medical disorders or for the adult with these disorders in other areas such as vocational training have been established and maintained in all countries. Such lack provides a conflicting message to the parents with learning disabilities but also makes it difficult for professionals in the field.

While it is difficult to determine how successful individual programmes have been because of the lack of available information, it is apparent that there are wide differences in services so that it is difficult to determine the success or failure of any programmes. These issues, however, are of critical importance and hinder comparability across programmes. Thus, to say that one programme showed success while another demonstrated failure cannot be determined until one examines each of the factors mentioned below.

These include:

— whether the programme was established as a result of litigation (resulting in heightened feelings within the communities); whether it had limited funds for a limited period (usually removed from another area of need and resulting in a sense of urgency as well as a sense of lack of commitment and permanence); or whether the programme was established as a result of an identification of need, with planning regarding goals and objectives, evaluation and funding.

— whether the programme was affiliated to or funded by a private or public organisation known for specific philosophical, theoretical, religious or ethical views or requirements which dictated the approach, as opposed to a systematic identification and addressing of each parental need.

— what the motivation of the parents was to attend (e.g. were they required to attend by a social service agency in order to maintain or to regain custody of child versus voluntary or recommended participation). Programmes in which parents were required or forced to attend would be expected to show less positive results than those in which parents attended voluntarily.

— what the requirement of parental achievement was while in the programme (e.g. attendance only as opposed to active involvement, including learning certain critical skills to a criterion).
— what, if any, kind and level of resistance were shown by service agencies and/or by parent groups to this type of programme.
— the approaches used (e.g. traditional early intervention strategies such as maternal interaction versus health care).
— the numbers of parents served (most have only a few mothers).
— the characteristics of parents (most have higher functioning parents but many have parents with additional difficulties such as emotional disturbance and/or an abusive or disturbed partner).
— the characteristics of children, if any, actually served. Most programmes only served parents with very young children or only involved the young child. A programme also serving older or all children would have very different experiences from those only serving babies.
— the actual services provided (was there actual intervention in all or in only a few areas of need or only co-ordination of services? It is essential to know this before one speaks of success or failure).
— the length of the programme (most limited their involvement to an hour); its frequency (most met weekly or even monthly); its duration (most lasted for only a few months) and its periodicity (few if any provided ongoing follow-up with additional training).
— the location of the intervention (there was a great deal of variability, with many based at centres with home visiting; those providing services in the home appear to be more successful for some aspects of child care, but providing a social environment for the mother at a centre offers friendship possibilities).
— whether the training was done individually or in groups.
— the type of outcome used (most programmes used singular maternal outcome measures such as absence of reports of abuse and only a few used multiple outcomes).
— the maternal outcomes used. A few programmes assessed maternal knowledge and skill, often focusing on mother–child interaction. Only a few examined specific health care skills or used child outcome measures such as physical and health status (i.e. head circumference, weight and height, immunisation record, accidents, nutrition).

NEEDS

With all of this, there are a number of needs that have to be recognised in order to adequately understand and address the complex issues surrounding parenting by people with learning disabilities. These include:

— the need for clarification of who comes within the definition of 'a parent with learning disabilities'.
— the need for definitions of and criteria for establishing what constitutes 'adequate parenting', 'adequate child care' and 'adequate child development and health status' (Select Congressional Panel for the Promotion of Child Health 1981).
— the need for agreed parent as well as child outcome variables (including health status).
— the need for other theoretical models about parenting given the changes in society (i.e. away from the model in which the need for outside help is seen as making a parent somehow less than competent, since we know that within society as a whole, *all* parents require some degree of support during their child's lifespan).
— the need for other educational models. It is clear that the traditional educational models that rely upon good verbal and reading skills are not appropriate for use with this population or for other parents with poor educational skills.
— the need for co-ordination of service delivery models. It is clear that parents with learning disabilities, just like many other people with special needs, require many varied and ongoing services. In order to maximise their abilities these services need to be co-ordinated through a single broker.
— the need for other service delivery models including residential models.
— the need for a model for public education and its implementation in this area.
— the need for a model for professional education and its implementation in this area.
— the need for commitment and continuity by agencies.
— the need for co-ordination between federal, state and local agencies, professional organisations and services agencies. At the state and local levels, this includes co-ordination between licensing agencies such that alternative living arrangements can be considered and implemented. In many American states the numerous regulations mean that it is extremely difficult to establish a group home in which both the mother/father and the child can live.
— the need for examination of activities for other parents with special needs.

RECOMMENDATIONS

There are a number of recommendations that can be made including:

A range of support models

It is apparent that traditional support and living arrangements are biased towards child removal when less intrusive and/or restrictive alternatives may be appropriate. Alternative support models need to be considered and developed along with criteria for parents moving from one level to another. This could range from total independence, which involves living by oneself without any outside concern or support, to living by oneself with some support, to living with another person or family while still having major child responsibility, to living with someone who has primary child responsibility and who may even have guardianship of the child and/or of the parent and finally to actual child removal and parental separation. This last may be either permanent or not.

Training

With the above suggested changes, it is apparent that there is a need for the examination of ways to ensure that such changes are considered, developed and implemented equitably and fairly across the nation and the effects of that implementation evaluated. Some of these needs are clear, including training for existing staff members of various social service, medical, educational and legal agencies as well as training being included within college and university curricula.

Technical assistance

There is a clear need for the establishment of technical assistance centres to help programmes in their development and successful implementation.

Research

At present, our state of knowledge is such that we can say that some, perhaps many, parents with learning disabilities are not only able to, but actually do, provide adequate child care. Now, however, the questions have become more specific and include: What are the predictors of adequate parenting by persons with learning disabilities?

What resources are needed? And what happens to their children? A focused research effort is needed to answer these as well as other questions including:

— when does any youngster become a parent and under what circumstances? Do the youngsters who attended classes for those with mental handicaps, for example, have children earlier than do those who attended regular classes or who attended classes for the emotionally disturbed? Do they have more children or fewer? Are their children normal at birth? When do they begin thinking about having a child? Who are the men in their lives? We have found, for example, that the fathers of the children are often limited in some way, frequently with an emotional disturbance rather than a learning disability.

— when and if they become parents, where do they have their children? What services are provided for them, and later for their child?

— when and how do they obtain services later?

— what criteria are used to identify those parents needing services at a later date and are those criteria valid?

— if and when the needs of parents are identified, what services are available and what more is needed?

— what supports are available for parents with learning disabilities? Are their own parents available? Church personnel? Others? Which supports do they use or not use and why? What methods can be employed to encourage uptake of supports?

— what preparation for parenting is provided in schools? Is education about what is involved in decisions of whether or not to become a parent available to these youngsters in special education?

— can predictors be developed to help prepare youngsters for parenting before they leave school? Can we predict those who are most likely to be parents before they leave school and provide additional help? If we can, what type of help would be optimal and how can it be delivered?

— what happens to the children of these youngsters in comparison to those of other youngsters?

— is the incidence of abuse and/or neglect the same for youngsters who have attended classes for those with learning disabilities as for those who attended other classes? Or is the incidence for abuse actually higher for others but the incidence of neglect the same?

— what are the public policy issues that need to be addressed in the short term as well as in the long term to address the needs we identify?

— what are the professional training needs for the legal profession? For other social service workers? For educators?

POLICY RECOMMENDATIONS

A recommendation is made that a two-pronged approach be used in systematically addressing the topic of parents with learning disabilities within the USA. A similar approach may work within the UK. Prong one should be ongoing and deliberative in order to garner support and to identify impediments and facilitators. At the same time, however, given the information that we already have available, a number of things should be implemented immediately as part of prong two.

At the public level

Members of the media should be brought together for information development and dissemination about this sector of the population.

At the federal governmental level

1 Co-ordination/Policy

Key people from each of the federal or national agencies should be brought together to:

— gather information regarding what each has done or is planning to do in this area.
— have an information presentation on this topic.
— become part of an Inter-agency Task Force to ensure co-ordination of federal or national efforts for this population.
— develop goals and adopt a plan of action to respond to these goals systematically.
— establish criteria for the acceptance of programme proposals (with reviewers being carefully selected to ensure they are familiar with this population).

The action plan should be shared with other governmental and non-governmental agencies at all levels but should specifically include private non-profit groups, foundations and professional organisations. The specific purpose of this sharing should be to increase co-ordination of efforts, to decrease the probability of overlap, to help to ensure that careful empiricism is followed and to hasten the build-up of information on this population.

2 The implementation of existing or new policies relating to this population should be ensured in:

— early intervention programmes
— public laws
— case management.

3 A tracking system for attainment of the agreed goals should be implemented.

4 Discussion and dissemination should be encouraged:

— presentations should be made on this topic at the meetings of service agencies and to the national conventions of each professional group.
— at the same time, public media should be invited and assisted to prepare stories on this topic.
— a number of manuals should be produced including one on how to develop and implement a service programme and one on policy decision-making for states/local government.

At the national non-governmental level

Similar efforts should be expended with national professional organisations.

At the state level

Information dissemination, co-ordination and data collection should begin with the agencies responsible for this population including schools, public health, the judicial system and social services.

Epidemiological and cost studies

There are urgent needs to determine how many parents with learning disabilities there are now and how many children they have, how many there will be in the future and what their needs are and what the costs will be to meet those needs.

CONCLUSION

As we have seen, the issue of parents with learning disabilities is an emotive one, both historically and currently. In this chapter we have proposed that we apply and build on the knowledge (as opposed to the opinions) we have of such parents and their parenting skills and needs in a systematic, co-ordinated manner. For this to happen in an optimum way, co-ordination at all levels of policy making, planning, service delivery, research and development is required.

ACKNOWLEDGEMENT

The authors would like to extend appreciation to the numbers of SHARE who have continued to provide support for this neglected area.

REFERENCES

Accardo, P. and Whitman, B. (1990) 'Children of mentally retarded parents'. *American Journal of Diseases of Children* 144, 69–70.

Bowden, J., Spitz, H. and Winters, J. (1971) 'Follow-up of one retarded couple's marriage'. *Mental Retardation*, 9, 42–3.

Brantlinger, E. (1988) 'Teachers' perceptions of the parenting abilities of their secondary students with mild mental retardation'. *RASE*, 9, 31–43.

Crain, L. and Miller, G. (1978) 'Forgotten children: maltreated children of mentally retarded parents'. *Pediatrics*, 61, 130–2.

Espe-Sherwindt, M. and Kerlin, S. (1990) 'Early intervention with parents with mental retardation: do we empower or impair?' *Infants and Young Children*, 2, 21–8.

Fantuzzo, J., Wray, L., Hall, R., Goins, C. and Azar, S. (1986) 'Parent and social-skills training for mentally retarded mothers identified as child maltreaters'. *American Journal of Mental Deficiency*, 91, 135–40.

Feldman, M., Towns, F., Betel, J., Case, L., Rincover, A. and Rubino, C. (1986) 'Parent education project II: increasing stimulating interactions of developmentally handicapped mothers'. *Journal of Applied Behavior Analysis*, 19, 23–37.

Garber, H. (1988) *The Milwaukee Project: preventing mental retardation in children at risk*. Washington: American Association on Mental Retardation.

Hayman, R. (1990) 'Presumptions of justice: law, politics and the mentally retarded parent'. *Harvard Law Review*, 103, 1201–71.

Lynch, E. and Bakley, S. (1989) 'Serving young children whose parents are mentally retarded'. *Infants and Young Children*, 1, 26–38.

Peterson, S., Robinson, E. and Littman, I. (1983) 'Parent-child interaction training for parents with a history of mental retardation'. *Applied Research in Mental Retardation*, 4, 329–42.

Ramey, C. and Campbell, F. (1984) 'Preventive education for high-risk children: cognitive consequences of the Carolina Abecedarian Project'. *American Journal of Mental Deficiency*, 88, 515–23.

Schilling, R., Schinke, P., Blythe, B. and Barth, R. (1982) 'Child maltreatment and mentally retarded parents: is there a relationship?' *Mental Retardation*, 20, 201–9.

Seagull, E. and Scheurer, S. (1986) 'Neglected and abused children of mentally retarded parents'. *Child Abuse and Neglect*, 10, 493–500.

Select Congressional Panel for the Promotion of Child Health (1981) *Better Health for our Children: a national strategy*. Washington: Superintendent of Documents, DHHS Pub. No. 79–55071.

Slater, M.A. (1986) 'Modification of mother-child interaction processes in families with children at-risk for mental retardation'. *American Journal of Mental Deficiency*, 91, 257–67.

Tymchuk, A. (1985) *Effective Decision Making for the Developmentally Disabled*. Portland, Oreg.: Ednick Communications. Republished Austin, Tex.: Pro-Ed Communications, 1989.

Tymchuk, A. (1990a) *Parents with mental retardation: a national strategy*. Washington, DC: President's Committee on Mental Retardation.

Tymchuk, A. (1990b) 'What information is actually found on labels of commonly used children's over-the-counter medications?' *Children's Health Care*, 19, 174–7.

Tymchuk, A. (1990c) 'Assessing emergency responses of people with mental handicaps'. *Mental Handicap* 18 (4): 136–42.

Tymchuk, A. (1991) 'Assessing home dangers and safety precautions: instruments for use'. *Mental Handicap* 19 (1): 4–10.

Tymchuk, A. (1992) 'Predicting adequacy of parenting by persons with mental retardation'. *Child Abuse and Neglect* 16, 165–78.

Tymchuk, A. (submitted a) 'Childhood illness symptom recognition, comprehension and treatment by parents with and without mental retardation'.

Tymchuk, A. (submitted b) 'Depression symptomatology in mothers with mental retardation'.

Tymchuk, A. and Andron, L. (1988) 'Clinic and home parent training of a mother with mental handicap caring for three children with developmental delay'. *Mental Handicap Research*, 1, 24–38.

Tymchuk, A. and Andron, L. (1990) 'Mothers with mental retardation who do or do not abuse or neglect their children'. *Child Abuse and Neglect*, 14, 313–23.

Tymchuk, A. and Andron, L. (1992) 'Project Parenting: child interactional training with mothers who are mentally handicapped'. *Mental Handicap Research* 5 (1): 4–32.

Tymchuk, A. and Feldman, M. (1991) 'Parents who are mentally retarded: a review of the research relevant to practice'. *Canadian Psychology* 32, 486–96.

Tymchuk, A., Andron, L. and Unger, O. (1987) 'Parents with mental handicaps and adequate child care – a review'. *Mental Handicap*, 15, 49–53.

Tymchuk, A., Andron, L. and Rahbar, B. (1988) 'Effective decision-making/problem-solving training with mothers who have mental retardation'. *American Journal of Mental Retardation*, 92 (6): 510–16.

Tymchuk, A., Hamada, D., Anderson, S. and Andron, L. (1989) 'Emergency training for mothers who are mentally retarded: a replication'. *The Mental Retardation and Learning Disability Bulletin*, 17, 34–45.

Tymchuk, A., Yokota, A. and Rahbar, B. (1990a) 'Decision making abilities of mothers with mental retardation'. *Research in Developmental Disabilities*, 11, 97–109.

Tymchuk, A., Hamada, D., Andron, L. and Anderson, S. (1990b) 'Home safety training with mothers who are mentally retarded'. *Education and Training in Mental Retardation*, June, 142–9.

Tymchuk, A., Hamada, D., Anderson, S. and Andron, L. (1990c) 'Emergency training with mothers with mental retardation'. *Child and Family Behavior Therapy* 12, 31–47.

Tymchuk, A., Andron, L. and Bavolek, S. (1990d) *Nurturing Program for Parents with Developmental Disabilities and their Children.* Park City: Family Development Resources, 7687 Buckboard Circle.

Tymchuk, A., Andron, L. and Tymchuk, M. (1990e) 'Training mothers with mental handicaps to understand behavioural and developmental principles'. *Mental Handicap Research*, 3, 51–9.

Whitman, B. and Accardo, P. (1990) *When a Parent is Mentally Retarded.* Baltimore: Paul H. Brookes.

12 Interventions with a pregnant woman with severe learning disabilities

A case example

Sandra Baum

Working with clients who have severe learning disabilities often presents us with new challenges which stretch our professional competencies, skills and therapeutic techniques, requiring us to work in unexplored territories with little documented advice. It came as a surprise and shock to a large residential unit for people with learning disabilities when a 24-year-old, non-verbal woman was discovered by the senior registrar to be 24 weeks pregnant, after the client had been complaining of pains in her stomach. We desperately wanted to proceed with the care of the woman in a way which accorded with our acceptance of the five accomplishments (O'Brien 1987) and our commitment to the principles of 'normalisation' (Wolfensberger 1972). We thus sought to adopt a professional, caring and responsible attitude to the situation.

This chapter describes a multidisciplinary team's involvement in the initial assessment of the situation and the issues involved, preparing the woman for the birth of her child during the last three months of pregnancy, the preparation for the grief of separation of mother and child and the subsequent interventions post-birth. Whilst not providing all the answers, it highlights the questions and complex issues raised by the interactions between the client and the staff groups and hopefully gives some insight into the role of the clinical psychologist as a co-ordinator and facilitator.

ASSESSMENT OF THE SITUATION

Psychological assessment

As a clinical psychologist, I became involved with Carol (not her real name) at the request of the psychiatrist who wished to ascertain the client's degree of learning disability and general level of functioning in order to support any recommendations should the case come to court. Carol's cognitive and intellectual abilities were difficult to assess, since many of the psychological tests available were age-inappropriate and not validated on adults. However, on the non-verbal Coloured Progressive Matrices test (Raven 1956) results indicated that she had an equivalent IQ of below 40. Legally this put her in the 'severely impaired' range of intelligence. A client who has an IQ of 54 or below is legally considered to be incapable of giving consent to sexual intercourse and thus the pregnancy could be judged to be the result of a criminal act (see British Psychological Society 1991, Gunn 1989).

Further evidence that Carol had severe learning disabilities in her social functioning was demonstrated using the Adaptive Behavior Scale (Nihira *et al.* 1975). Carol was described as being ambulant, doubly incontinent, requiring her to wear large incontinence pads, able to eat unaided and wash her hands and face, but in need of assistance with bathing. She was able to dress and undress without prompting but was very dependent on direct care staff in all areas of self care, being unable to look after her needs independently. Carol had no sensory disabilities but was practically non-verbal, only saying a few one-syllable words such as 'yes' and 'no'. She could use basic Makaton for her immediate needs, responded to facial expressions when she was spoken to and could understand basic instructions. She was able to name many pictures and concrete objects via the use of Makaton signing (Walker 1980) and was able to identify parts of her body. Carol was able to recognise familiar people and had an awareness of others, although she was described as a 'loner', only interacting in a passive way. She was not considered a management problem by the direct care staff but occasionally pulled at her hair when she was in distress.

Decisions to be made

Initially the unit's response to the situation was that of panic. The psychiatrist sought advice from various agencies including the Medical Defence Union, the British Medical Association's Ethics Committee and solicitors, whilst, as a clinical psychologist, I sought advice from other professionals in the field regarding the dilemmas we faced. It soon became apparent that the ethical and legal situation was far from clear. Because of the severity of Carol's learning disabilities, she was unable to provide informed consent to the termination of pregnancy. Since the Mental Health Act of 1983, a guardian can only consent to psychiatric treatment, and this 'has left a gap in the law whereby nobody can consent to an operation on a severely mentally handicapped adult' (Dyer 1987). The Medical Defence Union argues that doctors should not perform an abortion on a woman with severe learning disabilities without consent or sanction from the court. Thus the English law does not provide any satisfactory answers. With reference to the case of T (1987), the view held was that it is to be determined by the treatment provider whether the treatment is in the best interests of the patient's health and whether it is dictated by good medical practice. If these conditions are met, then the treatment provider can go ahead. But it was acknowledged that this was not entirely satisfactory. Thus we were in a very delicate position: the foetus was already 24 weeks by scan, being close to the legal limit for abortion, and medical, ethical and legal decisions had to be made urgently.

Multidisciplinary meetings were held including all key personnel involved in Carol's care plus her family to aid the decision process. Relations with the family were particularly strained; her relatives blamed the unit for not being vigilant, not supervising her 24 hours a day and, more importantly, asked why her pregnancy had not been discovered until such a late stage.

Three major issues were discussed. Was the pregnancy likely to be the result of a sexual act imposed on her? Could we recommend termination or should the pregnancy go to full term? What support would she need in whatever decision was made? Much multidisciplinary discussion centred on the circumstances of the conception. Carol was very much a loner, she was not known to have any relationships with men, often rejected the approach of others and did not like to be touched. Staff who had known her for over six years were shocked to hear that anyone could have got close enough to her to have engaged in sexual intercourse. She had never returned to the house in a distressed state or with any of her clothes or incontinence pads disarranged. However, there had been one incident where she had been missing for a period of time and found outside the unit's grounds. This did not coincide with the time of conception. We were left to conclude that in view of her history, it was likely that the sexual act had been imposed on her and that the perpetrator was someone that she knew well. Male clients, staff and relatives were thus under suspicion. In view of our conclusions, the Police Child Protection Team was asked to investigate the circumstances surrounding the conception.

With regards to the issue of termination, the team had heated discussions prejudiced by our own personal beliefs, but trying desperately to seek what was in Carol's best interests. Carol was unaware of her pregnancy and could not express a view regarding either its termination or continuation. We thus considered whether any woman would want to carry a foetus to term which may have been the product of abuse plus the delicate issues regarding the rights of the unborn foetus, which the scan and routine antenatal blood test indicated was normal. We also had to take into account the chances of the foetus being developmentally or physically handicapped (see Gath 1988) and the issue of babies with handicaps not being popular for adoption or fostering. Other issues discussed included the child being the subject of a care order at the time of birth and that Carol would not obtain any benefits from bearing the child.

In so far as support was concerned, it was evident that up until now the pregnancy had affected Carol negatively. She was pulling her hair out, she did not like carers touching her and resisted carers' attempts to bath her. Whatever course the pregnancy was to take, it was evident that Carol needed emotional and practical support. If the pregnancy was terminated, it would have to be done legally and quickly. She would need to be counselled and supported throughout this time. If the pregnancy was to continue, she would need to be prepared for the birth of her child, and to be allowed to grieve for the loss of the child due to immediate adoption. She would need to be treated in a dignified way, have a quiet and private living space and there would need to be close liaison with the obstetric team.

In spite of these lengthy discussions, the final decision was taken out of our hands: it would take too long for the case to go to court and our legal advisors were unable to give us clear guidelines. Second, we were unable to find an obstetrician and midwife team who would carry out a termination at this late stage. With much relief, the team began to discuss the preparation for the birth of Carol's child and the subsequent loss of the child through adoption.

The Police Child Protection Team

Since sexual abuse was suspected, we had a moral duty to call in the local Police Child Protection Team. Its investigation took the form of interviews with the client aided by the social worker and the clinical psychologist, interviews with staff members and male service users, family interviews and examination of written records kept on the house. The psychological assessment was very useful to them as it gave a picture of Carol's level of communication and an overview of her skills and degree of learning disabilities.

The Protection Team was very tactful and professional, taking care to interact with her as an adult rather than a child. With the aid of anatomically correct dolls and Makaton signing, Carol was able to reveal that she had had sexual intercourse with a man and that it had 'hurt'. She was in much distress and though unable to say conclusively who the man was, the police were satisfied that the conception had been the result of a criminal act. Further police investigations, however, resulted in inconclusive evidence and thus the case was closed.

PREPARATION FOR BIRTH

Over the next three months a core team of professionals, i.e. the clinical psychologist, senior registrar, direct-care staff, instructors from the social education centre and the social worker, met on a weekly basis to discuss guidelines for good practice regarding Carol's last three months of pregnancy. The main role of the team was to provide mutual support, to communicate with all personnel on practical management issues and to identify the specific roles of each professional so that no aspect of the pregnancy was overlooked. As a clinical psychologist, my role within the team was often to act as an information gatherer and facilitator. At the same time, I also co-ordinated all interventions with the client, acting at three levels namely: direct counselling and teaching Carol; staff support and liaising with the managers of the service to ensure that all her needs were met.

Initially, guidelines for good practice were discussed in the absence of any policy guidelines within the unit. Our approach was based on O'Brien's (1987) five accomplishments (community presence, competence, choice, individuality and respect), plus Craft's (1987) six sexual rights and values (namely the rights to grow up, to know, to be sexual, not to be at the mercy of the individual sexual attitudes of different care-givers, not to be sexually abused and the right to humane and dignified environments). Our guidelines focused on Carol's need for privacy; the need for her to be told that she was pregnant and that there was a baby inside her; the need for her to be taught about the stages up to the birth and the birth itself; the need for her to be allowed to grieve for the 'loss' of her baby; her physical needs and our liaisons with the obstetric team; the needs of the other residents on her house and staff support. The following sections describe in detail how the above guidelines were implemented and the interventions adopted.

Her need for privacy

The team members agreed that Carol needed privacy in her own environment. At the time, as is the practice in institutional care, Carol shared a bedroom with seven other women. Whilst this is not a suitable environment for any client, we acknowledged the necessity of Carol having her own room for rest and quietness, for this to be 'dignified', and with pleasant decoration, whilst not infringing on the rights of other women to remain in their own beds. Fortunately, a client was moving out of the house, back to her borough of origin, which vacated a bed in an adjoining two-bedded room. The manager of the service arranged for this room to be converted into a single bedroom (through the erection of a wooden partition). This was decorated and comfortably furnished. The less expensive option of moving Carol to another house which had single rooms was considered inappropriate as we did not wish to give her added stress or for her to feel punished or abandoned during this difficult time. Morale was high in the team after this work was completed, as we all felt that management was supporting us in our efforts to meet all of Carol's needs.

The need for Carol to be told that she was pregnant

Carol had the right to know what was happening to her body towards the preparation of birth and to be given as much information as she could assimilate. Thus the aims of this part of the intervention were to inform her that she was pregnant and that there was a baby inside her.

It seemed appropriate that this work should be performed by the instructors from the social education centre because they had known Carol for a number of years, they had teaching skills for working with clients individually and it was important for Carol to continue her day care for as long as possible. A core of three instructors met with myself to discuss interventions and the plans were shared with the direct-care staff. Unfortunately, we did not have access to *Not a Child Anymore* (Brook Advisory Centres 1987), *Life Horizons 1* and *2* (Kempton 1988) or similar materials. Also, many of the educational materials available from the local health education unit were much too complex or inadequate for clients with severe learning disabilities. Thus, we were forced to work with Carol using minimal resources and therefore had to be creative with our interventions. In retrospect, if these packs had been obtainable they would have been invaluable to the work we were doing. The clinical psychologist's role at that time was to advise on how and what interventions should be implemented; also, to repeat some of the work done with Carol at the social education centre in the evenings and during her days of non-attendance. The social worker informed Carol's relatives of the nature of our intervention in an effort to keep channels of communication open. This proved to be difficult, as relations with them were already strained because of the understandable blame they attached to the unit for us 'allowing' her to become pregnant in the first place.

Evidence from the psychological assessment indicated that Carol was able to point to different parts of her body and that she could name photographs of objects using Makaton signing or by pointing to concrete objects in her immediate environment. Thus, photographs and line drawings could be used to aid her understanding that she was pregnant. The instructor began by showing photographs taken during her own pregnancy, including pictures of her holding her baby immediately after the birth. She then showed Carol photographs of herself having a big stomach and touched Carol's stomach, saying, 'Baby in me in the photograph . . . baby in Carol'. We managed to obtain a book with simple coloured line drawings (Docherty 1986) showing a baby inside a woman's stomach, to help Carol understand that there was a baby growing inside her, and used these pictures daily to reinforce the message that 'a baby was inside Carol'. We were thus extrapolating two-dimensional photographs to the three-dimensional medium of Carol being pregnant, and we were concerned as to whether she was grasping this extrapolation. To ensure that she was understanding our teaching, we asked her questions such as, 'What is in your tummy?'. Carol would point to the picture of the baby in the representations and thus we had some indication that our teaching was proving successful. These were difficult concepts for Carol to comprehend, particularly as the concept of 'inside' is abstract and cannot be seen. However, we were confident that she understood the term 'inside' as this had been demonstrated in the psychological assessment with the use of the *Merrill-Palmer Scale of Mental Tests* (Stutsman 1948). We were conscious, though, of the necessity of using simplistic language to aid, rather than hinder, her understanding.

The need to be taught about the stages up to the birth

Carol was learning that the baby was inside her 'tummy', but the stages of pregnancy, the time factor involved and the idea of growth were difficult to explain. We briefly gave her an explanation of sexual intercourse to indicate why she had got pregnant using the pictures from the book, asking Carol questions such as, 'Why is there a baby inside you?', and Carol pointed to the picture of a man having sexual intercourse with a woman and pointed between her own legs. We did not concentrate on conception as we feared that this would be giving her too much information to assimilate and that the concepts would be too difficult to grasp. The instructor and myself faced many dilemmas on how much time we should give to the issues of sexual intercourse since sexual abuse had been suspected. We did not wish to distress Carol more than necessary or interfere with the Police Child Protection Team and its investigations. Also, we had limited time in which to prepare her for the birth and thus had to prioritise our teaching; we did not give her detailed information on parts of the body or the sexual lifecycle.

We had difficulty explaining the gestation time, the growth of the foetus and the change in her shape. We gave her a calendar highlighting approximately how many days and weeks it would be until the birth of her child and took photographs of her stomach from the side, sticking them on the calender each week to show her the difference. Second, we drew the outline of Carol's stomach each week on the same sheet of paper in an attempt to show her that her stomach was growing. Third, we used photographs to try and illustrate the growth and development of the foetus during pregnancy. We were very much working with uncertainties. We only knew approximately when the baby would be born, and thus we were trying to prepare her for a birth that could happen at any time. Also, we were uncertain that Carol was grasping these abstractions sufficiently due to her apparent lack of time concept and our difficulty of not being able to assess this adequately. We were working on the assumption that it felt more comfortable as professionals to give her the information as concretely as possible in the hope that she would understand some of the information, rather than assuming that she could not understand at all. Her visits to the maternity unit for her antenatal care would hopefully reinforce this counselling and give her a chance to see women at different stages of pregnancy. However, until she felt the contractions and with her case packed went into hospital, we had no way of knowing whether she knew when her baby was to be born.

During these last twelve weeks up to the birth of her child, we reiterated to Carol that, 'It is your job to look after the baby whilst it is in your tummy'. We did not go into details of how the foetus breathed or ate but said that she must sit down as much as possible, not carry her large bag around with her and eat lots of healthy food. Carol was able to do this successfully, possibly due to the fact that physically she was becoming very large and tired, and thus she used to rest for long periods of time.

Focusing on the delivery

Initially, we were working on the assumption that Carol would have a vaginal delivery since there was no physical reason to suggest otherwise. We introduced this by saying that, 'It is the nurses' and doctors' job to help the baby to come out of Carol'. We informed Carol that when the baby was ready to come out it would give her much pain and that this would 'hurt'. We found it difficult to explain to Carol how she could tell when labour started. Again, pain is an abstract concept until the person experiences it, and we were telling her that she would be in pain at some time in the future, but had no evidence to suggest that she was understanding this teaching apart from her facial expressions. Often when we talked to her about 'pain' she screwed her face up, showing us that she understood the concept but, more importantly, communicating to us her fears.

We used photographs and a video from the local health education unit showing the birth of a baby to explain the process of delivery. We initially introduced this with the sound turned down, as we were conscious that the images together with the sound might have been too distressing at the outset. We talked through the video with Carol and paused it at different stages. We assessed her understanding by asking her questions such as, 'Where will the baby come out?', and 'Who will help Carol to bring the baby out?'. Carol gave us the answers by pointing to her own body or pointing at the television screen. This work also included some explanation of the anticipation of pain to be experienced during the birth. We turned the sound up on the video to introduce her to the noises and facial expressions of the woman, informing Carol that she would feel pain and that it would hurt because the baby had to come out of a small space. Carol responded to this by contorting her face.

Liaison with the midwives was essential during this stage of intervention. They informed us which techniques Carol should learn to help her in the delivery room and we carried out the interventions with their regular advice and support. These included breathing techniques, bending and opening her legs and the use of the face mask for the inhalation of nitrous oxide and oxygen as a self-administered form of analgesia. With regard to breathing techniques,

Carol had to be taught the difference between short and long breaths to aid her through the labour. This was achieved by teaching her to regulate her breathing through the use of candles, tissues held in front of her mouth, perfume and 'breathing together' with the instructor or clinical psychologist. Within a week of introducing this, Carol was able to respond appropriately when asked to demonstrate a short or long breath. Carol was taught to bend and open her legs by lying on a mat in her bedroom with a towel resting on her thighs for modesty. She was given her face mask by the midwives to practise breathing with whilst at home. This was introduced at an early stage to desensitise her to the mask, as we hypothesised that she might be frightened if it was first used in the delivery room.

Carol made regular fortnightly visits to the antenatal clinic with direct-care staff. This was increased to weekly as the time got nearer to the birth. During these appointments, Carol visited the delivery room, labour, and post-natal wards to familiarise herself with these new environments. She also had the chance to see other women who were pregnant. We often repeated to Carol that when she went into hospital with her suitcase and when her stomach really 'hurt', she would be ready to have the baby with the help of the nurses and doctors.

We approached this part of the intervention with much apprehension. We were never sure, at any stage, whether the skills we were teaching her would adequately equip her for the confinement in hospital. The direct-care staff were unsure whether they could recognise the signs and symptoms of labour; and the multidisciplinary team were uncertain that she would be able to cope with a vaginal delivery, be able to lie down for long periods of time or cope with the contractions and the immense pain of labour. We were particularly concerned that, as Carol had been doubly incontinent for many years, she might not be able to use ordinary muscular control necessary for pushing and to aid the contractions. Added to this, would she be able to use breathing techniques taught in this stressful situation? Would she act 'destructively' when she was in pain? We shared our worries with the obstetric team, who were very skilled in allaying our anxieties, inviting two advocates to be present at the birth. (Details of our liaisons with the obstetric team will be discussed below.)

The need to be allowed to grieve for the 'loss' of her baby

Perhaps the most distressing aspect of all the interventions was to prepare Carol for the subsequent 'loss' of her child once it had been born. There was no question in anyone's mind that Carol could conceivably look after the baby, and thus Carol's social worker liaised with child social workers to arrange for immediate adoption. We could not ignore the fact that, whilst Carol had the right to know about all aspects of her pregnancy, she also had the right to know that she could not keep the baby and it would be taken away for someone else to look after.

We introduced these difficult concepts verbally, using simplistic language, trying to explain that she would not be able to look after the child, discussing this in terms of her own dependence on other people and comparing this to the baby's dependence. These ideas were presented to Carol by informing her that it was someone else's 'job' to care for the child. 'When the baby comes out, it will be another mother and father's job to look after it. Carol cannot look after the baby. Carol wears nappies, the baby wears nappies. Carol cannot talk, the baby cannot talk. Carol is looked after by the staff, the baby will be looked after by another mum and dad.' We discussed this with Carol in a positive manner by saying that it was 'good' that Carol was going to have a baby and 'good' that another mother and father were going to look after it, but we acknowledged the sadness and grief that Carol would feel when she said, 'Goodbye'.

We were conscious that in an effort to make the experience concrete and to aid the bereavement process, Carol would need to have a photograph of herself with the child; would need to be introduced to the adoptive parents; and that photographs should be taken showing her saying 'goodbye' to the child when it was given to the new parents. These recommendations were discussed with members of the obstetric team and they were happy to oblige with our requests.

Music therapy was also introduced at this stage and continued after the birth, as a means of exploring and understanding Carol's emotions in a non-verbal medium. The role of the therapist, then, was to develop a relationship with Carol, to understand, reflect and interpret musically therapeutic issues that were relevant to her.

At a subjective level with regards to our pre-birth teaching, Carol's facial expressions of sadness and anguish, her eye contact with her 'teachers' and, later, her actual crying, gave us enough feedback to convince us that she was comprehending some of the information that we were giving her. We were assuming that she would understand some of our simplistic language, but again, we were only giving her factual information as a way of minimising some of the trauma that she would face.

Other interventions

As Carol got closer to the time of the birth, her attendance at the social education centre ceased, due to her being given maternity leave. She spent long periods of time in the house, resting and sleeping in her bedroom. Obviously, she was becoming more uncomfortable physically during this time. To enable her to relax, we introduced soft music and used this as a medium for taking her through the 'fantasy' of birth and the subsequent separation from her child, often stroking her arm and hand. We also introduced aromatic oils into her bedroom to help Carol sleep or remain calm, and to refresh her. Lavender was used to promote calmness, and rose geranium because of its uplifting floral aroma and calming properties. Lemon, lemon-grass and orange oils were also used because they were refreshing. These oils were used to replace the familiar institutional smell. It was difficult to ascertain whether this technique had a positive effect on Carol in any therapeutic sense, but it did provide a more pleasant smell in her environment. Other techniques were employed including massaging Carol's back, neck and feet to help her relax.

Conclusions from the interventions used with Carol

Within a very short time of the interventions commencing, Carol's hair pulling, associated with distress, decreased. We hypothesised that her increased awareness of her predicament through teaching lessened this destructive activity. Carol was also experiencing a greater degree of one-to-one attention. It was apparent that she was enjoying the relationship with her 'teachers' and greater interaction from the direct-care staff. She was being praised and complimented, wearing new, bright maternity clothes and was made to feel special. All of these factors must have contributed towards these positive, observable signs. We were impressed and surprised by her apparent level of understanding and her grasp of some difficult concepts. This was evidenced by communicating with Carol via Makaton signing, gestures and her described behaviour. She was questioning our stereotyped beliefs that a person with an apparent IQ of less than 40, as judged by psychometric assessment, could not possibly gain knowledge or cope with extreme changes in her body. The immense progress and 'maturity' gained in her understanding encouraged us to continue with this intense level of social and practical support.

As professionals, we were concentrating on her rights as a woman, to be made fully aware of the situation regardless of her disability.

The assumption held was that information could be made comprehensible if it was given pictorially and by the use of simplistic language. We had an obligation to educate her about the predicament, to give her the necessary tools so that she could cope with the birth as best she could. The knowledge given was to allow her to take some responsibility, to help reduce the fear and distress, and this was the key to her being treated and valued as an adult.

Liaisons with the obstetric team

Liaisons with the local obstetric team at the District General Hospital were vital to ensure that Carol received the full antenatal care afforded to all pregnant women. The direct-care staff did not have any obstetric training and were anxious that it would be difficult to recognise signs and symptoms of labour, particularly since Carol was non-verbal and doubly incontinent. We were also concerned that Carol's 'emotional' needs would not be taken into consideration during her confinement. Thus communication and preparation were vital. Through direct contact with the midwives and by letters to the consultant obstetricians, we discussed our wishes for Carol antenatally, perinatally and post-natally, stressing the importance of the team getting to know Carol and being fully aware of our interventions as well as being given the psychological assessment of Carol's severe learning disabilities. Liaisons were led by the senior registrar and direct-care staff.

The obstetric team agreed to Carol being seen by the same midwives at her regular antenatal appointments and at the time of the birth. They showed her around the delivery room, the labour and post-natal wards, and gave her a face mask to practise breathing with whilst at home. She met other women who were pregnant during her visits to the hospital, and the midwives gave our team helpful and supportive advice in answer to any questions that were raised. All of these interventions helped Carol to familiarise herself with these new environments and 'uniformed' strangers, with the added benefit of somewhat reducing her fear and distress.

Our team was concerned about whether Carol could cope with a vaginal delivery and we shared our worries with the obstetric team, whilst simultaneously stressing that this mode of delivery should be allowed unless there were any physical difficulties. It was agreed that two advocates could be present at the birth and that sterilised mats and cushions could be used in the delivery room with the aid of soft music, to allow Carol to move around if lying down for long stretches of time became too stressful.

The obstetric team also had no objection to Carol being given her own private room in the maternity wing. Our reasons were that if the baby was going to be taken away from her immediately after the birth, it would be very distressing for Carol to be on a large post-natal ward and to witness other mothers with their babies. We also requested that she should stay in hospital for at least one week after the birth to convalesce. This was agreed if our unit could provide a member of staff throughout the day to keep her occupied, as the Maternity Wing had few staff able to provide this cover. We also discussed the necessity of Carol being allowed to hold the baby, to have photographs taken with the baby and to be able to say, 'Goodbye'. The midwives informed us about procedures connected to immediate post-birth management, particularly the baby having an initial breast feed to obtain colostrum, which contains immune bodies and vitamins, and also the suppression of lactation in Carol's breasts, which would be hard, heavy and painful. We were also told that the community midwives would visit Carol at home during the puerperium stage, which lasts up to eight weeks post-birth, to check on her recovery.

We were extremely grateful for the support given by the obstetric team. They were very caring and ensured that Carol obtained the same facilities as would be available to any other woman in pregnancy. They allayed many of our anxieties, and regular communication made certain that Carol's needs were met sensitively and were given the utmost priority.

The needs of other residents

The needs of other residents who lived with Carol plus those who attended the social education centre had to be discussed with the multidisciplinary team, particulary since, of necessity, Carol was receiving extra attention. Concern was raised that this might have led to adverse reactions towards her. This was difficult to overcome due to staff shortages which typify services for adults with learning disabilities. However, we tried to ensure that Carol's fellow residents were offered some extra attention by other members of staff informally. It was agreed that residents should not be told formally that Carol was pregnant, as ordinarily it is unlikely that any woman who is having her child adopted would want the information publicly shared. However, if residents asked individually they were told the situation honestly. Naturally, confidentiality was important as we did not want to gain unnecessary media attention, which would have created a further burden and would not have been in Carol's best interests. Thus discussion of the situation was kept to key personnel only.

Staff support

All the professionals involved with Carol's care had responsibility for giving and receiving support. As a team we had not experienced this situation before, and therefore it was vital that we could share our skills and concerns. As mentioned previously, confidentiality was essential and thus we could only discuss the matter with each other. The weekly meetings, then, were vital to ensure that all of Carol's needs were met. Members often felt like 'expectant fathers': we were excited by the prospect of the birth, worried about Carol's reactions and saddened that she could only spent a short time with the child. We learned a lot about each other's roles and gained respect for each other's professions. We were testing the practicalities of working in a truly multidisciplinary way with close liaisons between many statutory agencies. Without gaining respect for and trust in each other and working through differences of opinion, our own personal biases and beliefs, we could not have worked effectively towards the common goal of making this experience as minimally traumatic as possible.

THE BIRTH

In her thirty-eighth week of pregnancy, a pelvic X-ray revealed that, on medical grounds, an elective Caesarian section would have to be performed and so the necessary consent forms were signed. We had little time to prepare Carol for this. A few days before her admission, the instructor and myself tried to explain the procedure to Carol by Makaton signing, gesture and speech. We used the face mask to indicate that breathing into this would put her to sleep and then said, 'When you wake up, the baby will not be in your tummy anymore. You will be sleepy and it will hurt, so you will stay in hospital for a few days'. This preparation seemed so unsatisfactory. We suddenly had to ignore weeks of preparing her for a vaginal delivery and discuss a different mode without evoking any new fears of a 'doctor cutting her open'. Second, would she think that the baby was still inside her if she had not experienced it coming out? At the time, these issues remained unresolved. The direct-care staff prepared her for the event by packing the suitcase with Carol and talked to her about the familiar people she would meet in hospital.

It is perhaps fair to say that our team were relieved by the decision to perform a Caesarian section but pleased that it had been made on medical grounds only. Carol was safely delivered of a healthy 'normal' 8-lb baby. The obstetric team lived up to our expectations by meeting all of Carol's needs. The midwife met her at the entrance when she arrived and one of the direct-care staff was allowed to stay with her throughout the birth. We were also informed that Carol took the face mask voluntarily to breathe into in the delivery room!

After the birth, Carol saw her child on several occasions. This was an emotional experience for all concerned. Her gentleness and joy at seeing the baby and for the first time saying, 'Baby', filled us with pleasure and sadness. Twenty-four hours after the birth, the baby went to foster parents. Carol was able to say 'goodbye' by handing the baby over to its 'new' parents. Photographs were taken. The foster parents were very co-operative and sensitive to these wishes. Carol seemed exhausted and sad, her face filling with grief and anguish at this inevitable separation.

Unfortunately, this latter stage of the process was unplanned. The hospital social workers wanted the baby to be given to the foster parents as soon as possible and had made these arrangements without informing us of the time or day of this union. By chance, we found out about this rendezvous a few hours before it was due to happen and thus we were able to quickly arrange for Carol to see her child for the final time to go through the separation rituals. It had been our oversight not to have liaised with the social workers previously to share Carol's need to say 'goodbye'. We were angry at their view that because Carol had severe learning disabilities this ritual was unnecessary. In retrospect, we should have discussed our plans with them to have minimised confrontation.

POST-BIRTH

Carol remained in the maternity unit for five days after the birth. During this time, extra members of staff from her home sat with her for company and engaged in 'table-top' activities to keep her occupied. This was important since she was quite isolated in this single room. Carol was already beginning to feel restless and bored. It seemed as though she was getting tired of being stuck in one room and this situation had become her prison.

During the first few weeks post-birth, Carol gradually became her usual self. Physically, she recovered extremely well under the super-vision of daily visits from the community midwife and the district nurse. Emotionally, she was experiencing mood swings and having periods of crying. It was apparent to all who knew her that she was going through a process of bereavement for the loss of her baby and the extra attention that had decreased in intensity. Her anger at the loss was directed primarily towards the carer who had stayed with her throughout the birth. She displayed poignant behaviours such as kicking her carer between the legs and was particularly averse to any physical contact. Other 'angry' behaviours included stamping her feet and shouting. It was likely that Carol was associating the loss of the baby with the carer who had also been there when the baby went to the 'new' parents and was attaching the blame to her. This created a terrible strain on the carer. She had given up so much of her off-duty time for the welfare of Carol and had been so compassionate, having developed a deep attachment. The carer could not help feeling angry and 'let down' by this attack.

The issue of not receiving as much attention was also important. Carol had received so much input from the key professionals during the last twelve weeks to prepare her for the birth. Now we all needed time to reflect and to do other work that had been left. Necessarily one-to-one attention decreased. She still received music therapy but other interventions ceased. This obviously must have had an effect on her. She was not so special now, the situation was not so urgent and we had other clients to consider.

Carol was given a framed photograph of her new-born baby, which she put under her pillow. She was also given a photograph album depicting all the stages of her pregnancy and birth. It was important that we achieved some kind of balance and that we did not make the pregnancy the most significant event in Carol's life. To do this we added other, earlier photographs of her to give a context and to show her life had value before the current experience.

PROTECTION ISSUES

Major issues now had to be discussed regarding her future safety and protection. In the last twelve weeks we had centred on the preparation for the birth of her child, now we had to focus on the issue of suspected sexual abuse. Lengthy case conferences focused on supervision issues, contraception, self-protection strategies and other concerns. As a clinical psychologist, part of my role within these meetings centred on discussing future self-protective strategies for Carol. We agreed that she had coped extremely well with her pregnancy and had shown that she was able to learn facts about her predicament. However, it was apparent that she was sexually vulnerable, ignorant of sexual knowledge and her personal rights.

In the context of a sex education programme we thus needed to teach Carol strategies for keeping safe and that familiar faces as well as strangers might mean danger. The approach developed in books by, amongst others, Ann Craft (1987), Hilary Dixon (1988), contributors in *Thinking the Unthinkable* (Brown and Craft 1989), *Not a Child Anymore* (Brook Advisory Centres 1987) and *Life Horizons 1 and 2* by Winifred Kempton (1988) have been invaluable in developing our strategies, and this work is still ongoing. We are teaching Carol skills to empower her but can never be sure whether she could use them in a real, unsafe situation.

SERVICE ISSUES

Carol's pregnancy had raised awareness within the service for the need to broach the whole area of sexuality and people with learning disabilities. It had raised issues regarding their sexual vulnerability and the need to empower service users by giving them education and skills to offer some protection against abuse and exploitation. As a service, we needed to be proactive rather than reactive by developing a cohesive structure for promoting these issues. First, we needed to develop sexuality guidelines (see Craft 1987) which had to be supported by management. Second, we needed to have access to adequate resources; money for materials, training opportunities for staff to develop skills and competencies, and information on the law. In the present climate of financial constraints, meeting some of these needs presents us with new challenges.

In relation to sexual abuse, we needed to be more observant and vigilant by looking for behavioural signs. It was important to acknowledge that problem behaviours may develop as a consequence of abuse, rather than other factors, and thus we had to be cautious in just intervening from a behavioural perspective.

CONCLUSIONS

It is not very easy to draw clear-cut conclusions from this story, since much of the evidence presented is necessarily impressionistic. However, it does seem fair to record that the multidisciplinary team unanimously felt that, though Carol had severe learning disabilities, her experience of the later stages of pregnancy was not a negative one but rather involved constructive and developmental features.

Several implications follow from this observation. First, at a theoretical level, the case example presented suggests that classifying people with severe learning disabilities on the basis of an IQ label *alone* is unsatisfactory. For, within IQ ranges, at whatever level, there is considerable variance. As Clements (1987) states:

> The powerful administrative labels applied to people affected by severe learning disabilities have done much to overshadow their psychology and render difficult the study of the uniqueness of each individual.

Thus IQ is not the major psychological feature of the individual. Rather, interventions used in this study support the shift towards the more humanistic approach of 'normalisation' (Wolfensberger 1972), focusing on Carol's individual needs and meeting them in sensitive and creative ways according to her level of understanding. It can be argued that this approach is in direct contrast to the comments raised by the Law Lords in debating whether F should be sterilised or not (*F case* 1989). F was described as having 'the verbal capacity of a child of two and the general mental capacity of a child of four or five'. The Lords went on to say that: 'Because of her mental disability, however, she could not cope at all with pregnancy, labour or delivery, the meaning of which she would not understand. Nor could she care for a baby if she had one. In those circumstances it would, from a psychiatric point of view, be disastrous for her to conceive a child'. Although not all the circumstances surrounding the F case are known, it might be concluded from the present case example that, given enough support and teaching, even a woman with an IQ of below 40 can cope with pregnancy. Clearly the allocation of resources in terms of time, materials, creativity and compassion is the key issue. It may be always the case that 'severely mentally handicapped mothers will be unable to rear and nurture their children who will therefore be taken from them and placed elsewhere' (Gillon 1987), but it is not necessarily the end of the world if they do become pregnant. It does not have to be the most disastrous thing that can happen if we are willing to provide the right environment.

ACKNOWLEDGEMENTS

I would like to thank all my colleagues who worked with me throughout this case, particularly the House Manager, the Instructor and Senior Registrar. I would also like to express my gratitude to Ann Craft, Michael Gunn, Valerie Sinason and Vicky Turk who offered invaluable advice and support.

REFERENCES

British Psychological Society (1991) *Mental Impairment and Severe Mental Impairment: A search for definitions.* London: British Psychological Society.

Brook Advisory Centres (1987) *Not a Child Anymore: A Social and Sex Education Programme for Use with Young Adults with a Mental Handicap.* Birmingham: Brook Advisory Centres.

Brown, H. and Craft, A. (eds) (1989) *Thinking the Unthinkable: Papers on Sexual Abuse and People with Learning Difficulties.* London: Family Planning Association.

Clements, J. (1987) *Severe Learning Disability and Psychological Handicap.* Bristol: Wiley.

Craft, A. (ed.) (1987) *Mental Handicap and Sexuality: Issues and Perspectives.* Tunbridge Wells: Costello.

Dixon, H. (1988) *Sexuality and Mental Handicap: An educator's resource book.* Cambridge: Learning Development Aids.

Docherty, J. (1986) *The Royal Society of Medicine: Growing Up, A Guide for Children and Parents.* London: Modus Books Ltd.

Dyer, C. (1987) 'Consent and the mentally handicapped'. *British Medical Journal* 295, 257–8.

F Case (1989) in 'Re F; F v West Berkshire Health Authority, *The Times* 25 May.

Gath, A. (1988) 'Annotation: mentally handicapped people as parents'. *Journal of Child Psychology and Psychiatry* 29 (6): 739–44.

Gillon, R. (1987) 'On sterilising severely mentally handicapped people'. *Journal of Medical Ethics* 13, 59–61.

Gunn, M. (1989) 'Can the Law Help?', in Brown, H. and Craft, A. (eds) *Thinking the Unthinkable: Papers on Sexual Abuse and People with Learning Difficulties.* London: FPA Education Unit.

Kempton, W. (1988) *Life Horizons 1: The Physiological and Emotional Aspects of being Male and Female. Sex Education for Persons with Special Needs.* Santa Monica, Cal.: James Stanfield and Company.

Kempton, W. (1988) *Life Horizons 2: The Moral, Social and Legal Aspects of Sexuality. Sex Education for Persons with Special Needs.* Santa Monica, Cal.: James Stanfield and Company.

Nihira, K., Foster, R., Shellhaas, M. and Leland, H. (1975) *AAMD Adaptive Behavior Scale.* Washington, DC: American Association on Mental Deficiency.

O'Brien, J. (1987) 'A guide to life-style planning', in Bellamy, G.T. and Wilcox, B. (eds) *A comprehensive guide to the activities catalogue: an alternative curriculum for youths and adults with severe disabilities.* Baltimore, Maryland: Paul H. Brookes.

Raven, J.C. (1956) *Coloured Progressive Matrices (CPM).* London: H.K. Lewis.

Stutsman, R. (1948) *Guide for Administering the Merrill-Palmer Scale of Mental Tests.* Yonkers, N.Y.: World Book Co.

T case (1987) in 'Re T; T v T and another', *The Times* 11 July.

Walker, M. (1980) *The Makaton Vocabulary Language Programme.* Makaton Vocabulary Development Project, 31 Firwood Drive, Camberley, Surrey.

Wolfensberger, W. (1972) *Normalization: The Principle of Normalization in Human Services.* Toronto: National Institute on Mental Retardation.

13 Almost equal opportunities . . . developing personal relationships guidelines for social services department staff working with people with learning disabilities

David Fruin

INTRODUCTION

1971 was a significant year for people with learning disabilities. In April 1971, the Education (Handicapped Children) Act 1970 swept away the concept that some children because of their handicaps were incapable of being educated: no longer would children be denied local authority educational services because of mental or physical disabilities. The education of all children became the sole responsibility of local authorities and since then the value of the resources and of society's value of such children has gradually increased.

That same month saw the implementation of the Local Authority Social Services Act 1970 and the setting up of social services departments. These new departments merged the responsibilities of previously separate welfare, mental health and children's departments so that social services for children with learning difficulties were no longer split between two different local authority departments.

In June of that year, *Better Services for the Mentally Handicapped* was presented to Parliament (DHSS 1971). This important White Paper stated that future service developments should be led by local authorities providing small residential homes and hostels, not isolated like many existing hospitals but in the centres of population, with residents taking part in the life of the community. And in terms of changing people's values, 1971 was particularly significant for the setting up of the Campaign for the Mentally Handicapped with its commitment to values of 'normalisation' (even if the original title now seems dated).

These new responsibilities and new organizations, together with the *Better Services* document, were important in setting the direction and pace of new services and in encouraging better allocation of resources. Two decades later, a whole generation of children – and their parents – have grown to accept and expect levels of personal development and services way above those of twenty or thirty years ago. Such expectations extend to include issues of personal and sexual relationships.

EFFECTING CHANGE

Legislative and organisational changes are usually introduced to remedy operational deficiencies and working practices. Yet, resistance to change on the part of front-line staff and their immediate managers is frequently encountered. At the same time, those with experience of major change know only too well that the work and turmoil of implementation often mean that direct services with clients take a lower priority. New legislation will not necessarily effect immediate differences for clients: attitudes, skills and knowledge of front-line staff do not change overnight.

STAFF

Staff are the major resource in organisations like social services departments and considerable efforts are with them needed to ensure that policy changes are carried through into practice. Often little attention is given to the inertia of individual staff members and of groups of staff in terms of their attitudes. Stability of attitudes particularly occurs with working groups such as those of the police and teachers – the canteen and staff-room cultures – or in relatively closed communities such as long-stay hospitals, or old-style Local Authority hostels or day centres.

Where organisations have a fast turnover of staff, introducing new approaches may be relatively easy but, compared with many organisations, the turnover of local government employees is low. One consequence is that there are many people still employed, some in senior positions, to provide services for people with learning disabilities who started their careers before 1971 and have had to respond to significantly changing public and professional attitudes to and expectations of their clients.

VALUES

An added factor inhibiting change among staff who work face-to-face with people with learning disabilities is that most of these staff enter their first such job without prior specialist training. Values and attitudes influencing choice of employment thus assume greater importance than in settings where people first have to undergo some form of education and training which provide opportunities for the promotion of current ideas and policies.

The Jay Committee (DHSS 1979) noted that:

> The staff's attitude towards the questions of sterilisation and of whether to discourage or encourage sexual relationships amongst mentally handicapped people suggested that this was an area which presents them with difficulties. About 40 per cent of both groups of staff (ie. in hospitals and LA homes) felt that more mentally handicapped patients or residents should be sterilised.

However, a significant principle of the Jay Committee was that 'mentally handicapped people should be able to live in a mixed sex environment. For adults this would include the right and opportunity to get married'.

In practice, such new views had more impact in the local authority residential sector than in hospitals. Not only did the numbers of people living in local authority homes double from 1971 to 1981, while hospital numbers declined, but managers of new local authority hostels and homes did not have to battle with the active resistance to change shown by hospital nursing staff. In the hospitals, the scepticism of ward-level staff about their patients' potential for development and their doubts too about the services provided by Local Authorities was well evidenced in the conservative, even reactionary, response of many nursing staff to the Jay Committee's proposals.

Nevertheless, the Jay Report added impetus to the work of many specialist staff and middle managers developing new models of services, as exemplified in the King's Fund Centre's *Ordinary Life* document (1980). For example, hostel units were being desegregated so that men's and women's rooms would be on the same corridor rather than being reached by separate staircases. Adult Training Centres were losing their preoccupation with maximising output from industrial routine production work and instead becoming Social Education Centres, encouraging clients to develop off-site activities, often unsupervised by centre staff. As a consequence, staff were increasingly being faced with situations which could be seen as indicative of the success of ordinary-life principles: individuals were developing personal friendships, like other people of their age, which could be a prelude to a sexual relationship.

Conceptual and professional direction came from groups such as the Campaign for the Mentally Handicapped (CMH), the British Institute of Mental Handicap and the National Development Group, later to become the National Development Team. But with rare exceptions, there was much less of a lead from Directors of Social Services nor was there evidence of a groundswell of support from front-line staff.

For top management, the personal relationships of a specific group of clients do not demand strategic decisions about finance or resources. Moreover, these are issues where values and opinions can predominate, not necessarily amenable to influence by 'technical' facts. It is also a topic in which elected members, parents and relatives and the wider public could be expected to take a livelier interest than usual in council matters.

ABSENCE OF GUIDELINES

But where were the policy guidelines to aid practice? In the past, the overt and covert messages were in agreement: sexual behaviours should be discouraged, a view derived from the still lingeringly influential eugenics arguments and from the perception of adults with learning disabilities as being forever children, devoid, like idealised children, of any sexual feelings. Although the new policies and practices recognised that repression, easier to administer within the closed communities of long-stay mental handicap hospitals, was no longer appropriate, in the absence of a positive lead from top management, the policy by default became one of denial.

In organisational terms, this could only be a short-term solution since unit managers – especially officers-in-charge of homes – were the people who most experienced the conflict between the formal absence of a departmental policy and the practices on the part of their clients and of their staff. And it was this group of managers who would be most at risk of censure should some 'incident' occur.

DEVELOPING GUIDELINES IN HERTFORDSHIRE

In Hertfordshire, it was from such middle managers that pressure for a clear departmental policy led to the setting up of a guidelines working group. The Principal Officer (Mental Health), with managerial responsibility for mental handicap units, on taking up his post in 1985 soon found that almost all unit managers were anxious about 'skeletons in their cupboards', i.e. clients' interpersonal relationships which more senior managers were unaware about, and for which no guidance to support staff practice was available. In January 1986, he obtained agreement to set up a working group to explore the possibility of developing staff guidelines on the sexuality of people with learning disabilities. At about the same time, evidencing the changes occurring on a nationwide basis, other social services departments and voluntary agencies, e.g. Avon, Barnet, Brent, Camden, Hereford and Worcester, Hounslow, Mencap Homes Foundation (1987) and MacIntyre Homes, were also embarking on similar exercises.

By July of that year, the Hertfordshire Working Group was able to submit an initial draft to the Director but the work of the Group was soon overtaken by a major departmental reorganisation. It was not until 1987 that the work was revived and the task of redrafting the guidelines allocated to the new Development Officer responsible for services for people with learning disabilities.

In Hertfordshire, as elsewhere, the task was made easier by being able to draw on previous published documents including the guide and review material authored by Craft and Craft (1981, 1982). One document which had a wide influence was Paul Chamberlain's King's Fund Centre publication (1984), *Personal Relationships and People with Mental Handicap*, not only because of its substantive content but also because its publication by such an influential organisation was able to legitimate for sceptics the validity of open discussion of such sensitive issues. Another helpful document was an exploration of the legal position (Gunn and Rosser 1985).

However, for organisations such as social services departments it is usually not enough to import a ready-made document and adopt it wholesale: organisations and their staff need to work through for themselves the ideas and adapt the procedures to conform to the house-style of other policy and procedure documents and, more importantly, in order to develop a sense of ownership towards the finished product. This was certainly true for Hertfordshire.

The Development Officer undertook an extensive round of consultation with staff groups, enabling the draft guidelines to be checked out against case examples and modified. These discussions also provided the opportunity to raise both individual cases and general issues, and thus acted as a form of in-service training.

Eventually, a further draft was approved in summer 1988 by the department's senior management team for circulation to other council departments and to members of the county's four joint planning teams for mental handicap services. Again, modifications were made in the light of feedback.

GETTING COUNCILLORS' APPROVAL

Because of the sensitivity of the topic and the need to ensure that elected members shared in the new and overt statement of policies and procedures, the decision was taken that the guidelines should be presented to councillors for their endorsement. In September 1988, a report seeking approval of the department's proposals was presented to the Social Services Community and Care Sub-Committee, with the draft guidelines included as an appendix. At that time, although the Conservatives were the largest group, none of the three major political parties had an overall majority on the Council. At the Sub-Committee meeting, co-opted members from the voluntary sector spoke strongly in favour of the draft guidelines, as did speakers from the Labour and Liberal Alliance groups. The Conservative members were more cautious and expressed some disquiet about the guidelines, tabling a resolution proposing that three elected members and the Director of Social Services should review the issue and report back to a future meeting of the Sub-Committee. In the event, the proposal was defeated and the Sub-Committee recommended to the main Social Services Committee that the guidelines be adopted.

The debate caught the attention of the local press, with headlines such as 'Row over sex guide', 'Mentally ill to get sex talks' and 'Taboo sex under council spotlight'. Councillors were lobbied by a number of groups, including the East Hertfordshire CMH group. At the Social Services Committee meeting in October, again the debate was lively and for the most part split on party political lines. The recommendation for approval was only passed on the casting vote of the Labour Chairman of the Committee so that under the Council's standing orders the report had to go forward to the next full meeting of the County Council. At this meeting, the voting strength of the Labour and Alliance groups was sufficient to resolve that the guidelines be adopted as formal County Council Social Services policy.

CARRYING THE GUIDELINES INTO PRACTICE

Following the Council's endorsement, the guidelines were published in booklet form, distributed widely throughout the department and made available for public sale (see appendix). Since that time they have also served as the basis for a series of training courses held regularly since 1988. Such training has involved staff attending one-day off-site courses as well as sessions at individual residential and day centre locations. Without the follow-up of training, the impact of such published procedural material would be considerably reduced.

One of the fears of some staff and observers, prior to publication of the new guidelines, was that parents would be over-protective and deny the personal and sexual needs of their adult sons and daughters. In fact, once staff began to raise these issues for debate, most – but not all – parents were keen and indeed relieved to discuss their children's needs and behaviours in an open manner with residential and day centre staff. The printed format of the publication, available free to all such clients and their families, could serve as an agenda for discussion and demonstrate that these concerns were not just applicable to their sons and daughters but were shared by others too. But the difficulties of embarrassment and the usual taboo nature of frank discussion about one's own and others' sexual and personal relationships showed that experience and training, particularly in the form of role play, were helpful in decreasing the tensions around these topics.

ABUSE

The changing climate within the department, the less restrictive policies towards clients and the continuing media publicity about child sexual abuse together have meant that staff, and perhaps clients and families too, are increasingly able to acknowledge the occurrence of abuse involving the department's adult as well as child clients.

Staff in almost every residential and day unit can cite present or past cases where abuse or the possibility of abuse or exploitation has been present. As with the general topic of personal and sexual relationships four years previously, no formal guidance was available. A working group was formed to develop procedures where physical or sexual abuse was suspected. The issuing of guidelines for staff has taken longer to achieve since the focus has widened to include all vulnerable adults who may be considered to be at risk.

THE PRINCIPAL FEATURES OF THE HERTFORDSHIRE GUIDELINES (Appendix)

Values

The values which underpin the policy guidelines are based on the widely accepted ordinary-life principles, together with an explicit recognition that risk cannot be excluded from individuals' personal, social or sexual lives. In addition to these general principles, there is also a more focused acknowledgement that people with learning disabilities are people with personal and sexual feelings and desires, and that as adults they are not children but people who, with rare exceptions, are not constrained or restrainable in legal terms from the types of social and personal relationships which people without learning disabilities engage in.

Departmental responsibility

A key feature of the guidelines is that individual staff members should not work with clients in an isolated way but their actions need to conform to and be supported by the department's policies and procedures. Risk, for example, needs to be shared with and justified to colleagues and managers and in this way the department is responsible from the top down for staff actions. Of course, this explicit sharing of responsibility is not limited to clients who have learning disabilities, but the guidelines aim to alter previous practice of front-line staff turning blind eyes or covertly supporting clients' sometimes dubious activities. In the past, clients' personal relationships and sexual matters in particular were taboo subjects which could not be discussed officially with senior staff and hence no endorsement for staff actions could be obtained. The department's publication of its guidelines clearly recognises personal and sexual issues as ones which its staff at all levels must face. Staff training and development play a critical role in bringing about changes in staff attitudes and social work practice.

Sharing and recording

One of the clearest statements in the guidelines is that individuals must not act alone but must share information with colleagues and managers. Another clear guideline is that staff, when preparing individual programme plans, need to review explicitly their clients' personal, sexual and interpersonal development and their needs for sex education. There must also be full recording. This is to ensure that these topics form an integral part of all plans which the department develops with and for its clients and do not get deliberately or inadvertently overlooked. These features of the guidelines are particularly important because as in most departmental casework there can be few general prescriptions about specific individuals' care plans. Thus, what does become of general significance is the *process* which department staff must follow to arrive at recommendations.

One of the few very specific proscriptions is a ban on intimate or sexual relationships between staff and clients, a guideline drawn to reflect the department's explicit statement of policy arising from a case a few years earlier where such a relationship had formed in a residential home for people of another client group.

CONCLUSION

The sexual and personal relationships of any individual – whether with learning disabilities or not – are too important to be omitted from any overview of an individual's life or to be denied and repressed. To deny or to attempt to hide the sexual needs, drives and feelings of people with learning disabilities is to repress a significant element of their personalities and to retreat to regarding them as second-class citizens. In today's world, this is no longer acceptable. But ensuring that front-line staff turn these principles into practice requires agencies to make a visible commitment to principles. They do this by publishing written guidelines developed locally to ensure their ownership at all levels of the organisation and then subsequently working through the implications with staff, clients and carers.

The Hertfordshire experience provides a useful model of turning rhetoric into reality.

REFERENCES

Chamberlain, P. (1984) *Personal Relationships and People with Mental Handicap*. London: King's Fund Centre.

Craft, A. and Craft, M. (1981) 'Sexuality and Mental Handicap'. *British Journal of Psychiatry*, 38, 494–505.

Craft, M. and Craft, A. (1982) *Sex and the Mentally Handicapped: A Guide for Parents* (Revised edition). London: Routledge & Kegan Paul.

DHSS (1971) *Better Services for the Mentally Handicapped*, Cmnd 4683, London: HMSO,

DHSS (1979) *Report of Committee of Inquiry into Mental Handicap Nursing and Care* (Jay Committee), Cmnd 7468, London: HMSO.

Gunn, M. and Rosser, J. (1985) *Sex and the Law* (2nd revised edition), London: Family Planning Association Education Unit.

Hertfordshire County Council Social Services Department (1989) *Departmental Policies and Guidelines for Staff on the Sexual and Personal Relationships of People with a Mental Handicap*. Hertford: Hertfordshire County Council.

King's Fund Centre (1980) *An Ordinary Life – Comprehensive Locally-based Residential Services for Mentally Handicapped People*. London: King's Fund Centre.

Mencap Homes Foundation (1987) *Staff Guidelines on Personal and Sexual Relationships of People with a Mental Handicap*. London: Royal Society for Mentally Handicapped Adults and Children.

Appendix

Departmental policies and guidelines for staff on the sexual and personal relationships of people with a mental handicap

Hertfordshire County Council Social Services Department

1989

PREFACE

Why is it necessary to produce guidelines on sexuality and personal relationships involving people with mental handicaps? That is a perfectly reasonable question. In many respects it would have been easier to have ignored the issues and avoid possible embarrassment. But to do so, although more comfortable, would be to fail people with mental handicaps, their carers and the staff who work with them.

In times past, many people with mental handicaps did not survive into adulthood and those who did so mostly lived in large isolated institutions. Nowadays, because of improved medical and social care, their life expectancy is similar to that of non-handicapped people. Furthermore, the pursuit of the policy of care in the community has resulted in the majority of those with severe learning difficulties living in domestic surroundings either with their own families or in hostels or group homes. The practice of 'normalisation' and 'integration' has offered new horizons to individuals with a mental handicap and enabled many to achieve their full potential.

For a growing number, life is no longer solely about needs, but is also about opportunities. Many will never have been in hospital except for the usual range of medical care and most will outlive their parents. A fuller life brings with it new experiences and some degree of risk. It is of importance that everything is done to reduce the danger of exploitation of vulnerable people.

The reason for these guidelines is to set out in clear terms the philosophy and practice of care and support for people with mental handicaps in order that they can be helped to lead a fuller life, with proper care and without the danger of abuse. The guidelines are explicit because to be otherwise would avoid tackling many matters which are often of the greatest concern.

Because the guidelines are radical and break new ground for Hertfordshire, we will be keeping them under review. We therefore welcome comments on their value.

I am pleased to have been invited to contribute in this minor way to the document because it affords me the opportunity to congratulate the authors, the individuals with mental handicaps, the parents and the staff who have contributed to its production, along with the Hertfordshire County Council who welcomed its publication. I have no doubt that it is a document which will be of great assistance to many and protection to others. I warmly commend it.

Herbert Laming
Director of Social Services

CONTENTS

INTRODUCTION

1. The Social Services Department provides services and works with many people in Hertfordshire who have mental handicaps. From time to time, staff are called upon to deal with and advise on situations, many of them complex, which involve the personal and sexual relationships of people with mental handicaps.
2. The Department has a responsibility to its staff and clients to provide guidance for those who work in this field, in order to encourage the development of responsible working practices and a county-wide consistency of approach.
3. Sex is a sensitive topic. Where the sexuality of vulnerable groups of people, such as children and individuals with a mental handicap, is being considered, then the topic is a particularly sensitive one, liable to arouse strong feelings and, sometimes, conflicting views. Because it is such an important issue, an agency such as the Social Services Department with its responsibilities for the welfare and development of vulnerable people cannot regard sex simply as a taboo topic, best ignored and forgotten until a crisis occurs.
4. Instead, and especially in the field of mental handicap, the Department needs to promote a positive and proactive approach aimed at ensuring that sexual matters are seen in the broader context of individuals' social and personal relationships. If this objective is to be achieved, the Department must present clear guidelines for staff who have care responsibilities for clients. Such guidelines can also serve as the basis for discussion with clients, their families and staff from other agencies.
5. The purpose of this document is therefore:

    A. To state the *philosophy* underlying the Department's *policies* on sexuality and people with a mental handicap;
    B. To specify Departmental *procedures* which should be followed in carrying out these policies;
    C. To discuss major *practice* issues; and
    D. To outline ways in which the *personal development* of individuals with a mental handicap and the *professional development* of staff can be fostered in this area.

    A Bibliography provides references.
6. This document has been developed in collaboration with staff working in the Social Services Department and other departments

of the County Council, with staff from other agencies and with representatives of voluntary and parent groups. It is, however, a Departmental document.

A. DEPARTMENTAL PHILOSOPHY AND POLICIES

1. Three broad principles underpin the Department's strategic philosophy in the field of mental handicap:
   - (a) People with a mental handicap have the same human value as anyone else and so possess the same human rights, with responsibilities.
   - (b) People with a mental handicap have a right and a need to live like others in the community.
   - (c) Services must recognise the individuality of people with a mental handicap.
2. Acceptance of these three general principles means that policies need to be developed in respect of sexuality which acknowledge that people with mental handicaps are just as likely to be born with sexual needs, drives and feelings as the population at large. Guidance for staff is needed to assist them to deal openly with what is acknowledged to be an area of considerable social sensitivity. Simply to deny or attempt to hide the sexual needs, drives and feelings of people with mental handicaps would be to repress a significant element of their personalities and to treat them as second-class citizens. Their individual sexual needs must therefore be considered within the wider context of their social and personal relationships. For example, when considering clients' Individual Programme Plans, their sexual needs and development should be covered. Such reviews should not assume automatically that people with mental handicaps cannot take on the responsibilities of sexual relationships, but should consider how they can be helped to cope with as many responsibilities as they are able and desire.
3. On the other hand, a major form of work with this client group must be to protect those who cannot take on full responsibilities and to guard against their exploitation and abuse. In any case, staff must ensure that plans and actions take place within the boundaries set by the law. And, in the same way that people with a mental handicap have the right to expect to live like other people, they also have the responsibility, as far as they are able, to act within the law and within the social constraints of the wider community.
4. If the Department is to encourage its staff to develop plans and

take actions involving the sexuality of clients with a mental handicap, then the Department has a responsibility to make explicit the guidelines which staff should adopt when taking decisions in this area. The Department must also recognise that, for some individual staff members, guidelines could support activities running contrary to their own personal views. However, as professionals, staff will be expected to refrain from imposing their own personal standards upon clients and to cooperate fully in team decisions.

5. Indeed, one of the reasons behind a key feature of the Department's guidelines – that all decisions about developing plans concerned with clients' sexual behaviours should be made within a team context – is to ensure that the views of a single staff member are not imposed upon individual clients. At the same time, staff will not be expected to undertake any illegal activity nor to condone any such activities.

6. It is against this background that the following statements are intended to summarise Hertfordshire Social Services Department's policies about sexuality and people with a mental handicap:

   People with a mental handicap should:

   a. be given the opportunity to express themselves sexually if they wish, in the same way as non-handicapped people;
   b. be protected from exploitation and abuse;
   c. be provided with education and guidance to assist them in their sexual development;
   d. be given opportunities to develop close, intimate, loving relationships; and
   e. have privacy which those relationships may require.

7. These policies do not imply that any particular expression of sexuality is to be imposed in blanket fashion on all clients with a mental handicap. People with a mental handicap, just like other people, vary considerably in their own attitudes and expectations regarding sexuality. Because of this, there can be no hard and fast rules for dealing with individual cases: staff will be expected to deal with clients and situations with sensitivity and care and to ensure that people with a mental handicap are free, if they so wish, for sexual matters to play a minimal role in their lives.

8. The approach to be adopted by staff towards the sexual development and behaviour of people with a mental handicap is part and parcel of the broader philosophy of 'normalisation' or 'ordinary life'. This philosophy leads to the adoption of policies which aim to reverse the devalued position previously taken by much of society towards people with a mental handicap by integrating them

more closely into the community in order to enhance the overall quality of their lives. In the past, considerable emphasis was placed upon attempting to develop risk-free, sheltered environments – asylums in the better sense of the word. An 'ordinary life' philosophy entails a shift from a primary focus on protection to the development of environments and experiences which allow a greater degree of personal choice and of privacy. However, an environment which allows greater degrees of personal choice and privacy can never be entirely risk-free. Such a consequence needs to be recognised by the Social Services Department and its staff and to be communicated to others, e.g. elected members of the Authority, the general public, other professionals and to clients and their families.

9. **Implications for the Social Services Department** In later sections of this paper, it will be apparent that many of the implications of the Department's policies relate to changes in attitudes and behaviours on the part of staff. However, there are also resource implications if these Departmental guidelines are to be carried forward effectively and these are discussed as they arise. For example, individual rooms should be the norm, fees may be needed to pay for outside specialist consultants, more case conferences may be required, etc.

10. **Training** If changes are to be achieved in care practices, one area which will be significant and to which additional resources will need to be allocated is training. Currently, the Training Section provides introductory study days and a 4-day course on personal and sexual relationships of people with a mental handicap. Part of the latter course focuses on developing programmes for providing sex education for adults with a mental handicap. In addition, discussion of sexual issues should take place as part of local induction training for new care and field staff arranged by line managers.

11. **Liaison with other County Departments and other agencies** Since social services for both children and adults with a mental handicap are often provided in close cooperation with those of other agencies, it is important that a coherent and consistent approach towards sexual issues be developed in liaison with staff from other agencies. In particular, the Education Department's policies towards the teaching of sexual and other personal and social topics need to prepare their pupils for the adult settings to which they will graduate. As a requirement of the Education Act 1986, special schools are designing new health education programmes, to

include sex education. Similarly, because of the close operational links which social services have with the health service and the need to seek specialist health, psychological and medical advice on sexual matters, it will be helpful if joint policies and practices can be agreed between Hertfordshire Social Services Department and the four District Health Authorities. The four Joint Planning Teams for Mental Handicap Services will be the appropriate fora for initiating discussions of these and related issues.

B. DEPARTMENTAL PROCEDURES

When considering issues relating to the sexual development and behaviour of clients with a mental handicap, the fundamental principle to guide staff of Hertfordshire Social Services Department is that *the practice objectives should be to maximise the clients' personal development*. But staff must also ensure that the behaviours which they seek to encourage are both lawful and socially acceptable.

1. Linked with this principle is the important basic guideline for practice that, as for other major issues in clients' lives, decisions about planning for a client's sexual and personal development, should not be taken by single staff members on their *own*. All clients, especially those for whom the Department has residential care responsibilities or for whom the Department provides day services, should have these needs considered in a case conference context to develop plans for Social Services staff, as well as clients themselves, their families and staff of other agencies. Such case conferences may include formal inter-agency Individual Programme Planning, Departmental reviews or supervision sessions but an essential requirement is that where decisions are taken these are recorded in writing. Agreed plans can thus be open to peer review and to line management approval.

2. *Individual staff should not take planned action which falls beyond the agreed and recorded plans, developed within a shared case conference setting.* In this context, the client's keyworker and linkworker have particular responsibilities, not only in terms of shaping the plans so that they take due account of the views of the client, parents, relatives, staff and other appropriate individuals, but also in communicating them to people who have a need to be informed. (A 'keyworker' is the person who co-ordinates on behalf of the department, the work with the client. A 'linkworker' is the person within a particular residential setting, who works with the client and links with the key workers.)

3. Such case planning will wherever possible and appropriate *involve clients and their families* as part of the decision-making procedure. In most cases, there will be a consensus about the plans for an individual's future. However, there will be occasions when the considered decision of the responsible Departmental professionals involved may conflict with the wishes of others with an interest in the individual's welfare. In such cases, (which will often highlight the independence and autonomy needs of clients) where the reasons for the decisions are explicit, recorded, have the backing of Departmental management and are taken in the best and long-term interests of the client, then these decisions should be implemented by staff.

4. Since both the development and execution of plans with an explicit sexual component may require skills routinely unavailable in the Social Services Department, it will be important to *involve other professionals with special skills,* where appropriate. Such professional skills may include those of the pyschologist, the family doctor, the nurse, staff working within a health education department or family planning agency or other specialist consultants. (In some cases, fees may be required to pay for such specialist consultants.) Where children and young people are concerned, it will almost always be necessary to involve Education Department staff.

5. Case planning involves anticipating and trying to shape the future. However, front-line residential, domiciliary and day care staff are often faced with situations which require immediate action and resolution. Staff cannot always wait until a case conference has been convened, deliberated and decided. As in other areas of their clients' lives, staff need to be informed about the plans developed in respect of sexual matters for their clients, so that staff actions can attempt to conform to the plans previously agreed. But *where immediate decisions must be taken which fall outside plans, staff will need to make their professional judgements in the light of the circumstances prevailing,* with the expectation that they will err on the side of caution, giving priority to the client care and protection responsibilities of the Department. In general, but particularly where sexual issues are concerned, it will be important for staff to report and record promptly what they and their clients have done. Such a procedure has the double value of protecting both client and staff members from possible later misunderstandings.

C. PRACTICE ISSUES

1. The legal framework
2. Personal and sexual development
3. Parental involvement
4. Bodily development
5. Masturbation
6. Petting
7. Sexual intercourse
8. Contraception
9. Sterilisation/vasectomy
10. Cohabitation and marriage
11. Parenthood
12. Unwanted pregnancy
13. Homosexuality
14. Pornography
15. Sexually transmitted diseases
16. Protecting clients
17. Staff relationships with clients

1.   The legal framework

1.1   People with a mental handicap are bound by and protected by the same civil and ciminal laws as other people. There are also special laws whose aim is to provide additional protection from exploitation and abuse for people with mental handicaps.

1.2   Men or women who have a state of arrested or incomplete development of mind, which includes severe impairment of intelligence and severe impairment of social functioning, are regarded in legal terms as 'defective'.

1.2.1   Section 7 of the Sexual Offences Act 1956 makes it an offence for a man to have unlawful sexual intercourse with a 'defective' woman.

1.2.2   In this context, 'unlawful sexual intercourse' refers to sexual intercourse outside marriage. A man would not be guilty of such an offence if he did not know and had no reason to suspect that the woman was a 'defective' for the purposes of action under the Sexual Offences Act.

1.2.3   Section 1(3) of the Sexual Offences Act 1967 prohibits a man from committing buggery or gross indecency with a 'defective' man.

1.2.4   According to Sections 14(4) and 15(3) of the Sexual Offences Act 1967, a 'defective' man or woman cannot give consent which, for any other person, would prevent any act from becoming an indecent assault.

1.2.5 Section 9 of the Sexual Offences Act 1967 makes it an offence for a person to procure a 'defective' woman for the purposes of unlawful sexual intercourse.

1.2.6 The term 'defective' as used here in the legal sense, is one which is limited in application. It is ultimately for a Judge and Jury to decide whether, in a case being heard before them, a person is guilty of an offence involving someone who is 'defective'. There is no procedure which can formally determine, in advance of such a court case, whether or not someone is 'defective' for the purposes of the Sexual Offences Act.

1.3 Under Section 128 of the Mental Health Act 1959, it is an offence for a male employee or manager in a hospital or nursing home to have unlawful sexual intercourse with a woman receiving in-patient treatment or with such a woman receiving out-patient treatment on the premises. Similarly, it is an offence to have unlawful sexual intercourse with a woman to whom a man is guardian or is in his custody or is in accommodation covered by mental health or social services residential accommodation or is a resident of a private or voluntary residential care home.

1.4 In general, acts which aid and abet others in the commission of offences, including those summarised above, are also offences.

1.5 Most people who are clients of the mental handicap services would not be regarded as 'defective' and are not therefore subject to these special restrictions and protections. Only if someone has *severe* impairment of both their intelligence and social functioning should they be categorised as 'defective'. Thus, the majority of social services' clients with a mental handicap could engage with others in sexual activities without those other people necessarily being at risk of prosecution.

1.6 It is therefore very important to consider the effects of classifying people with mental handicaps because, apart from the usual important concerns about the negative effects of labelling, classification has significant implications for the range of permitted sexual activities which an individual might wish to engage in. If staff of the Social Services Department believe that someone does have severe impairment both of intelligence and social functioning, and could therefore be regarded as 'defective' under the Sexual Offences Act 1956, then they should be aware that it would be an offence for someone to engage with that person in any sexual activity outside marriage.

It would also be an offence to aid and abet someone to engage in such activities.

1.7 Conversely, if Social Services staff wish to support one of their clients to engage in some form of sexual activity with another person, then it must be that they believe that the client would not be classifiable as 'defective'.

1.8 Staff will not be expected to undertake activities nor to support others in taking actions which are illegal. Whilst some staff may feel that the law in this area is unnecesssarily restrictive, the aim of the law is to protect vulnerable people and the Department will not support illegal actions on the part of its staff.

1.9 Because of the stigmatising and inappropriately enduring effects of labelling, the Department would not wish to encourage unnecessary categorising of clients. Discussions about whether or not to regard someone as 'defective' in the legal sense, would be expected only to arise for clients where the possibility of sexual relationship is being actively considered. Because people change, any consideration of someone as 'defective' should be periodically reviewed.

1.10 Where further clarification about legal issues is required, the County Secretary's Department should be consulted.

2. Personal and sexual development

2.1 People with a mental handicap have a right to develop personal relationships with other people. In some of these relationships there may well be a sexual component. This should not surprise us since the pleasures to be derived from sexual activities form a very basic part of us all. In the past, sexual feelings or behaviours exhibited by people with a mental handicap were often strongly discouraged by relatives or others charged with care responsibilities. Such suppression, and sometimes denial, were part of attitudes linked to eugenics or derived from a view of people with a mental handicap as eternally children, who ought to be devoid of sexual feelings. It is now recognised and accepted that people with a mental handicap do have sexual feelings. A responsible professional approach looks at sexual development as part of a wider concern to fulfil the potential of all clients, subject to working within the law and bearing in mind the impact of individuals' behaviours in a broader social context.

2.2 Thus, behaviours, such as masturbation in public areas of residential homes, should be discouraged because it is a criminal offence and appears to provide people with a mental handicap with a set of expectations which would not be acceptable for other people: carers need to educate their clients about the need to distinguish between behaviours which are and which are not acceptable in different places. Masturbation itself should not be discouraged but clients need to be taught that such an activity should only take place in private. On the other hand, for couples to hold hands or kiss is widely acceptable: people with a mental handicap should not be discouraged from such appropriate interpersonal behaviour just to maintain the stereotypes of some members of the public who might frown on public displays of affection between people with a mental handicap.

2.3 One consequence of teaching that some activities should only take place in private is that the Department and its staff need to enable people with a mental handicap, like others, to have the opportunity and the physical space, e.g. their own rooms like the rest of us, to engage in activities which most of us wish to do from time to time in private.

2.4 More generally, we need to take account of individuals' friendship patterns and to support these where there are mutual benefits. On the other hand, it is the professional duty of staff to discourage exploitative relationships and to ensure that people who do not wish to have enforced ties with others are not forced to do so.

2.5 Many people who come from the long-stay hospitals have suffered a life-time of broken relationships with other patients and with staff forever moving on. Staff in residential homes should be encouraging stable and long-lasting relationships and be discouraging casual relationships which can end by people being deeply and lastingly hurt.

2.6 In many cases, staff will need to take into account the religious and ethical views of clients and their families and these may differ between different ethnic and religious groups.

2.7 **Staff views** For carers of people with a mental handicap, just as for parents, education about sex is not something which can always be neatly packaged into pre-arranged time-slots. Staff need to be ready to respond to questions and situations as they occur. Sex should not be treated as something which is intrinsically bad and therefore a taboo or secret subject. Not all staff find dealing with sexual matters easy and supervisory staff must be aware of colleagues' difficulties in this area. Where staff have special difficulties, perhaps because of their own attitudes, they may need additional counselling or training to help them relate to clients in a professional way rather than simply on the basis of their own personal views. Some staff may hold strong views derived from their personal, moral, religious or cultural values. If these cause conflict with a Departmental decision about a course of action for a client, then these staff will need to discuss such conflict with their line manager to ensure that a Departmental plan for a client is not put in jeopardy.

2.8 **Sex education** Sex education counselling needs to be carried out on both an individual and group basis. Informal information-giving about sexual, as well as other topics, forms part and parcel of everyday work with clients, whether in a home or in a day centre setting. In day centres, there will also be value in providing scheduled sessions dealing in a more structured way with sexual matters. Making arrangements for these sessions is part of the responsibility of day centre managers. In general terms, sex education should be considered as part of a client's normal developmental process. However, teaching about personal and sexual development, whether for people with a mental handicap or for others, arouses in many people strong and conflicting feelings, sometimes derived from ignorance or our own embarrassment. On occasions, it may therefore be sensible to seek the advice and assistance of specialists such as SPOD (The Association for the Sexual and Personal Relationships of the Disabled), the FPA (Family Planning Association) or medical, psychological and nursing advice. For children and young people, it will be particularly important to ensure that the information and guidance being provided from the education services is in accord with that from the Social Services Department.

3. Parental involvement

3.1 Wherever relatives have close and active links with clients or the Department, it is good practice to involve them in case planning but there will be occasions when the views of the client and those of the professionals concerned with an individual's planning may differ from those of relatives. (In fact, such disagreements may more often arise over matters other than those to do with personal relationships.)

3.2 During 1987, the four Hertfordshire Joint Planning Teams for Mental Handicap Services each developed strategies which made reference to the individuality of people with a mental handicap. They also referred to situations where the views of those providing services to individuals might conflict with the views of relatives. In practice, especially where clients are children or where they live at home, it is more likely that the views of relatives, especially parents, will prevail. But as people with a mental handicap achieve independence and separation from their families, it is a measure of the extent to which they are regarded as *sons and daughters rather than lifelong children*, that their own views and those providing them with professional services will prevail rather than those of their parents and other relatives. In particular, where clients live away from their families, it will be inappropriate for all decisions to be automatically referred to relatives and such decisions may concern personal and sexual development and behaviour.

3.3 The guideline for practice as to whether or not to involve relatives in decisions about personal and sexual matters, as for other issues, will be the views of the Department's professionals as they consider what is in the best interests of the client. In respect of sexual and personal matters, it is important that such a decision should be shared by staff and recorded on the case file.

3.4 **Advocates** On some occasions, staff will wish to consider whether to involve someone who could serve as an advocate for a client, particularly where there is no direct involvement of relatives or friends.

3.5 Because sexual and personal development and relationships are such sensitive issues, there will be value in holding workshops for clients, relatives and staff which include presentations and discussions led by speakers from organisations such as SPOD or the Family Planning Association.

4.　Bodily development

4.1 Where the Social Services Department is responsible for the care of children with a mental handicap, carers and managers will need to liaise with the schools, the child's doctor and the health service to prepare children and their carers for the bodily changes of puberty which form important milestones in sexual development. Young people with mental handicaps often have less opportunity for learning from their schoolfriends about sexual matters than do their less handicapped peers: thus, the role of staff is especially important in providing this type of information and in encouraging respect for one's own and other people's bodies. Girls will need to be prepared for the onset of menstruation; staff may need to ensure that towels or tampons are changed regularly and that bathing and washing takes place to assist with hygiene. Boys will need to be informed about their own bodily changes and reassured about erections and the occurrence of wet dreams.

4.2 Intimate contact with clients, for example, when helping with personal hygiene or when giving assistance in bathing, should be by members of staff of the same sex. Where this is not possible, it is preferable that another member of staff should be involved to provide cover, or failing that, a more able client of the appropriate sex may be able to assist.

5. Masturbation

5.1 The sexual exploration of one's own body is a normal part of development and as such should not be discouraged. Masturbation is normal sexual behaviour for boys and girls and for men and women. However, people should be discouraged from masturbating in public places; staff should not convey the message that masturbation is intrinsically wrong but rather that it is socially unacceptable in certain places but acceptable in private places. If people seem to masturbate excessively, the reasons need to be discussed with other staff to decide on a course of action. The value of masturbation as a release from sexual frustration or tension should also be borne in mind.

5.2 Some people may need guidance to learn to masturbate successfully; decisions on such guidance clearly need to be shared ones and recorded. On some occasions, people with multiple handicaps may need physical aids to masturbate and staff may need to seek advice from organisations such as SPOD and the FPA.

6. Petting

6.1 The sexual exploration of other people's bodies is also a normal part of development but an activity which is constrained by social mores. People with a mental handicap should not be more constrained than other people simply because they are handicapped. However, there are circumstances when such behaviour is socially unacceptable or inappropriate and staff will need to assist clients to discriminate where and when intimate exchanges of affection are appropriate. The age, ability and degree of maturity of the clients will also affect what is acceptable behaviour and how clients should be advised. Staff need to take care not to convey directly or indirectly that all touch and exploration is wrong but rather that its expression may need to be limited in certain circumstances.

7.   Sexual intercourse

7.1 People with a mental handicap have the right to sexual relationships so long as they can give meaningful consent and such activities are within the law and take place in private. As indicated [on pages 255–7], if someone's social functioning is not 'severely impaired', even though they may suffer from a severe impairment of intelligence, it will not be against the law for another person to have sexual intercourse with them, providing consent is given. It is an offence for staff of residential homes provided for people with a mental handicap to have sexual intercourse with a resident.

8.   Contraception

8.1 Advice on contraception should be provided within an overall counselling programme where the relative benefits and disadvantages are discussed with the person concerned. Where a client is becoming involved in a heterosexual relationship, staff have the responsibility to be prepared to intervene to try to ensure that unwanted pregnancies do not occur. Clients should be assisted to make informed decisions in the light of advice obtained from their general practitioner or family planning clinic. (Some health authorities, e.g. East Herts, offer a specialist family planning service.) Such advice will be very much an individualised matter and no one should be forced to accept a particular method or any method. Whether or not to involve parents will be a subject to be considered with other professionals and the client herself or himself. Decisions will need to be shared ones and recorded on the client's case file.

9.   Sterilisation and vasectomies

9.1 In a rare number of cases, the possibility may be raised of sterilisation or vasectomy. This would be very much a last resort, for consideration after all other options have been examined and rejected. In view of the legal complexities where sterilisation or a vasectomy is being actively considered, the Area Director should be notified and advice sought from the County Secretary's Department.

10. Cohabitation and marriage

10.1 In today's society, there are few barriers to people deciding to live together as couples without being married. It would be inappropriate to place more hurdles in the path of people with a mental handicap considering such a step. However, staff need to advise potential couples about the long-term and the short-term implications of such a move, particularly in terms of impact on residential arrangements. A case conference should be called to endorse the plans for staff action. Where marriage is being considered, it will often be sensible at an early stage to involve a minister or other denominational advisor. The advice of the County Secretary's Department should be sought if there is doubt about the degree of mental handicap being such as to call into question the issues raised within the Matrimonial Causes Act 1973, i.e. the capacity to give consent or the ability to carry out the duties and obligations of marriage.

11. Parenthood

11.1 People with a mental handicap have the right to become parents but this right must be counterbalanced against the rights and needs of children. As indicated in the first principle presented [on page 250], with rights come responsibilities. Clients who express a wish to become parents will need counselling to explore their expectations and to assess their parenting capacities. Deciding to have children is an important decision for everyone, not just for people with learning difficulties. A positive decision to support or advise against someone with a mental handicap attempting to become a parent should be endorsed by a case conference.

12. Unwanted pregnancy

12.1 Where clients with a mental handicap are becoming involved in a sexual relationship, staff have the responsibility to be prepared to intervene and act to avoid an unwanted pregnancy. The client should be counselled about birth control and the implications of a sexual relationship. A decision to support a client in having sexual intercourse should be linked with a recommendation about the form of birth control which should be used. The advice of the client's medical practitioner or family planning clinic should be sought and the issue discussed and agreed by a case conference.

12.2 Should an unwanted pregnancy occur, clients should receive counselling on the options: the continuation of the pregnancy and the consequences for the baby's care; adoption; or abortion. Where a client is living in the residential care of the Social Services Department, the Area Director should be informed who will decide whether the advice of the County Secretary is to be sought.

13. Homosexuality

13.1 Lesbian activities and homosexual activities between consenting men over the age of 21 are not illegal. Homosexual behaviour involving a man under the age of 21 is illegal. Where adult clients have made a clear decision to engage in a lesbian or gay relationship, then staff should respect and support them in their personal and social development, provided they do not support behaviour which is against the law.

13.2 Attraction to members of the same sex can be a normal stage of development. Staff need to distinguish between normal exploratory behaviour during development, which may take place later in someone with mental handicap, and homosexual behaviour of an adult kind to avoid inappropriate labelling.

13.3 When considering the behaviour of clients engaging in homosexual behaviour, staff need to be sure that clients are not living in a setting where outlets for relationships with people of the opposite sex are restricted.

14. Pornography

14.1 Many adult men and women are interested in material which others would regard as pornographic. An interest in such material can be seen as part of the usual process of growing up, especially where the opportunity of open discussion of sexual matters is limited or suppressed. Where clients with a mental handicap have such material, possession should not be viewed in a less tolerant light than would be the case for people without a mental handicap. However, staff may find it useful to indicate that such material can give a distorted image of sexuality, can be degrading and can be offensive to other people. Where people living in Social Services accommodation possess pornographic material, they should be encouraged to keep it in their own rooms and out of sight, such material may offend others, for example domestic staff. People may feel discouraged from entering a room where pornography is displayed.

14.2 Staff should not promote the introduction of pornographic material into Social Services establishments.

15. Sexually transmitted diseases

15.1 Although as a group, people with mental handicaps are less at risk from sexually transmitted diseases, it is important that they are both appropriately informed about, and protected from, sexually transmitted diseases. As with the rest of the population, ignorance about the facts of transmission and of the effects of the diseases themselves will be widespread; staff will need to take advantage of informal opportunities to give information, but clients and staff themselves will benefit from formal instruction in this area. This will be a topic to be included in the sex education programmes which are provided in the day centres.

15.2 Where a client has a sexually transmitted disease, advice on working with such a client should be sought from the client's GP, with consent, and/or from health authority staff. Separate, Department-wide guidance is available for working with people with AIDS, of whatever client group. Guidance on Hepatitis B is also being formulated.

16. Protecting clients

16.1 The Department and its staff have a duty to protect clients who may be vulnerable to exploitation, although where clients can give meaningful consent to activities, then their wishes should be respected. In some cases, where staff are aware of the likelihood of exploitation or abuse, then there may be resource implications, e.g. to provide additional night cover in hostels. Staff need training to be alert to and recognise signs of sexual abuse.

17. Staff relationships with clients

17.1 From time to time, staff may develop strong attachments to clients and vice versa. Staff are employed to provide professional support to clients and such a relationship is essentially an unequal one. Where staff feel that their relationship with an individual client is going beyond that of a professional relationship, this is something which should be discussed with their supervisor. The Department cannot support any intimate or sexual relationship between staff and clients. If, after discussion with their supervisor, a staff member would wish to continue a relationship beyond that which would be permitted to an employee of the Department, then the staff member should consider resigning and thus having the possibility of developing a relationship outside that of staff member and client.

D. THE PERSONAL DEVELOPMENT OF PEOPLE WITH A MENTAL HANDICAP AND THE PROFESSIONAL DEVELOPMENT OF STAFF

1.   The personal development of people with a mental handicap

1.1 Sexual development, learning and behaviour should not be viewed in isolation from other aspects of an individual's development. Indeed, a rigid isolation of sexual issues from other matters, whether in terms of formal instruction or the informalities of everyday life, is likely to cause problems at a later date. Formal aspects of sex education, both in schools and in the Department's establishments will form part of a broad education programme covering such matters as health, hygiene, personal relationships, public and private behaviour, ethical issues, etc. Because of the individuality of children and adults with mental handicaps, a single programme will not usually be applicable for any one group of children and clients. In addition, staff will need to be sensitive to the varying interests and capacities of their clients.

1.2 For Social Services staff, probably more important than formal courses of instruction, will be their informal, day-to-day encounters with clients which will be influential in conveying knowledge and shaping clients' own attitudes about sexual matters. In general, staff should attempt to answer residents' questions openly, so that sexual matters are not dealt with in a secretive way. This is not an easy task to undertake professionally when so often in our own lives we are not able to deal with sexual matters in a straightforward fashion. The role of training for staff is important here, if staff are to be enabled to carry out such tasks in a professional manner.

1.3 From time-to-time, managers of residential and day establishments will need to review their programmes of activities to consider whether formal presentations of sexual issues need to be included in their establishments' programmes both for clients and for staff. In addition, staff with responsibilities for specific clients, e.g. caseworkers, keyworkers and linkworkers, when considering the individual programme plans of their clients, will need to review explicitly their clients' personal, sexual and interpersonal development and their needs for sex education.

2. The professional development of staff

2.1 In a number of places, this document has referred to the importance of staff's professional knowledge, skills and attitudes. The Department has two broad methods to ensure that staff employed by the Hertfordshire Social Services Department have the necessary qualifications in this critical aspect of personal and social life.

2.2 *At entry* into the Department's employment, managers will need to assure themselves that the staff they recruit possess positive and open attitudes to sexual matters. Once employed, many staff may require specific *in-service training* to equip them with more advanced and specialist knowledge and most staff, particularly those in face-to-face dealings with clients, will require occasional refresher courses on dealing with the sexual issues raised by clients with a mental handicap. Managerial support and supervision of staff – not only of front-line social workers but others such as domestic staff, escorts, etc – will be needed to provide continuing awareness of the issues of sexuality and personal relationships. Given the close collaboration with staff from other agencies, in-service and refresher courses could well be undertaken with staff from other agencies. In addition, short courses which include relatives and clients as course members as well as staff will be valuable.

2.3 Therefore, the Department should include, within its basic in-service training programme for all staff who work with people who have a mental handicap, at least the following types of training activity:
1. Study days on these guidelines and their implications.
2. A 4-day course on Sexuality and Personal Relationships for staff who would benefit from looking at these issues in order to feel more comfortable in their work with clients. Part of the course

would focus on developing programmes and course content for providing sex education for adults with a mental handicap.
3. Area groups should be established to consider dissemination and training needs arising from the adoption of these guidelines.

BIBLIOGRAPHY

Carson, D. (1987) 'The law and the sexuality of people with a mental handicap', edited proceedings of a conference at University of Southampton.

Craft, A. (1987) *Mental Handicap and Sexuality: Issues and Perspectives*. Tunbridge Wells: Costello.

Craft, A. and Craft, M. (eds) (1983). *Sex Education and Counselling for Mentally Handicapped People*. Tunbridge Wells: Costello.

Dixon, H. (1986) *Options for Change: A Staff Training Handbook on Personal Relationships and Sexuality for People with a Mental Handicap*. London: Family Planning Association.

Dixon, H. and Gunn, M. (1985). *Sex and the Law: A Brief Guide for Staff Working in the Mental Handicap Field*. London: Family Planning Association Education Unit.

Greengross, W. (1976) *Entitled to Love*. London: Malaby Press.

Mencap Homes Foundation (1987) *Staff Guidelines on Personal and Sexual Relationships of People with a Mental Handicap*.

MIND (1982) *Getting Together: Sex and Social Expression for Mentally Handicapped People*.

ORGANISATIONS

The Family Planning Association,
National Office,
27 Mortimer Street,
London W1

Telephone 071–636 7866

Sexual Problems of the Disabled – SPOD,
286 Camden Road,
London N7

Telephone: 071–607 8851

Name index

Subject index